GRADUATE MEDICAL EDUCATION
Issues and Options

GRADUATE MEDICAL EDUCATION
Issues and Options

Frank C. Wilson, MD

Foreword by
David C. Leach, MD

Radcliffe Publishing
Oxford • New York

Radcliffe Publishing Ltd
18 Marcham Road
Abingdon
Oxon OX14 1AA
United Kingdom

www.radcliffe-oxford.com
Electronic catalogue and worldwide online ordering facility.

British Library Cataloguing in Publication Data

A catalogue record for this book is available from the British Library.

ISBN-13: 978 1 84619 378 1

Typeset by Pindar NZ, Auckland, New Zealand
Printed and bound by Cadmus Communications, USA

Contents

Foreword

Residency is an intense experience; there is no steeper learning curve in medicine. The difference in skill and knowledge between interns and chief residents is profound. Residents are on a journey to become authentic physicians in which they discover both clinical wisdom and themselves. It is a journey that is surrounded by external drama, but which actually proceeds from the inside out. It is a journey that calls on the intellect, but also the will and the imagination. Residents learn to discern the truth, and to make clinical judgments in ways that are sometimes creative and even beautiful. It is the reason they went into medicine. It is a time when the habits of a lifetime are developed.

Frank Wilson has written an important book about this most formative time in a physician's life. In doing so he creates an opportunity for reflection about the history of graduate medical education, the key issues that consume present interests of medical educators, and the options that the profession and society have for going forward. His book offers information, insight, and inspiration about graduate medical education. It is timely. Workforce shortages, financial constraints, new knowledge and technologies, and dramatically changing demographic patterns in society pose challenges to graduate medical education. Changes are needed; will wisdom or reflex reactions inform the changes?

Dr. Wilson brings four decades of thought and experience as both a medical educator and practicing orthopaedic surgeon to this topic. He is reflective and has spoken and written about his experiences. Importantly, he writes well. Years of teaching undergraduate literature courses at the University of North Carolina have given him an affection for and skill with words.

How residents are taught, how they are evaluated, how their educational programs are funded, these and other critical issues are described in the book, as well as suggestions for their resolution. This work challenges us to be both effective and faithful stewards: effective teachers arming residents with the attitudes, skills, and knowledge needed to help patients in the new and emerging world, yet also faithful to the values and ideals of the profession. The great reforms in medical education of 100 years ago established a system of education that was both effective and faithful. Now that system is being challenged beyond its capacities. A new system is emerging that will be held to the same standards of effectiveness and fidelity. Lacking is clarity about the details of the emerging system; however, this book moves us closer to clarity and describes possible and thoughtful emerging solutions. It challenges us to think not only strategically but ethically as well. Dee Hock has said that we usually ask three questions when we should ask four.° The first three: Where have we been? Where we are now? Where we might be going? are covered; however, Dr. Wilson asks the fourth question as well: Where *ought* we to be going? Given the various vectors in play, what is the right thing to do to preserve our duty to the public?

Although he does not shy away from the major policy issues that need to be addressed, one gets the sense that his motives are not just expedient – he wants to preserve the goodness of the past into the future, while being malleable as to form and structure. He is driven by values and engages a creative, dedicated mind shaped by experience and a deep appreciation of the profession's obligations to serve the task.

° Hock D. *The Birth of the Chaordic Age*. San Francisco, CA: Berrett-Koehler Publishers, Inc.; 2000.

His effort reminds me of a poem by William Stafford, entitled: "The Way It Is."

The Way It Is

There's a thread you follow. It goes among
things that change. But it doesn't change.
People wonder about what you are pursuing.
You have to explain about the thread.
But it is hard for others to see.
While you hold it you can't get lost.
Tragedies happen; people get hurt
or die; and you suffer and get old.
Nothing you do can stop time's unfolding.
You don't ever let go of the thread.

William Stafford[†]

This book enables us to be more clear about the thread. It gives us something to hang onto as we "go among things that change."

David C. Leach, MD
Executive Director Emeritus
Accreditation Council for Graduate Medical Education
Asheville, North Carolina
August 2009

[†] Stafford W. *The Way It Is: new and selected poems*. Saint Paul, MN: Graywolf Press; 1998.

Preface

Were Flexner alive today, he would likely be making notes for another book dealing with the graduate aspects of medical education, which, still in the process of being born, did not merit mention in his 1910 landmark text. Medical school, though in need of reform, was preparation enough for the practice of medicine. The existence of 8500 residency programs encompassing 127 specialties and subspecialties would, a century ago, have seemed preposterous.

The need for more attention to education and university ties would doubtless appear again among Flexner's prescriptions for change, along with interdisciplinary linkages to care for patients with multiple and multifaceted diseases; and he would probably applaud the emphasis on performance and outcomes and the focus on residents as learners rather than helpers.

Medicine can be justly proud of the improvements in health care resulting from the labors of Flexner and others in the vineyards of medical education; but prospects for further progress are clouded by changes in the climate and soil of the vineyards themselves. The interplay of social, economic, and political forces will have a profound impact on the education of physicians and on the quality and delivery of health care.

My first thoughts for the preparation of this book revolved around revision of previous essays and papers on GME and organizing them as a compendium of work on what has been the keystone of my professional life. But it was not to be that simple.

Movement in GME prior to 1985 was largely academic and specialty specific: content and duration of training, guidelines for recertification and subcertification, and credentialing were issues for resolution within the house of medicine. Since the mid-1980s, influences outside of medicine, fueled by explosive population growth, social concerns, and technology, have become dominant players, threatening the foundations of the educational bridge between student and practitioner. An expanding and aging population, and the panoply of therapeutic options produced by innovations in science and technology has created overriding problems of access and cost, shortages that were compounded by managed care and the soaring costs of liability insurance. As physician reimbursement for each unit of service shrank, clinical "throughput" replaced the academic focus in teaching institutions, and in the rush to cure, care was almost forgotten. Treatment trumped empathy.

Clearly, the center had not held. With traditional values replaced by modern functionality, the very ethos of medicine had changed, for which more than an update of in-house issues was needed.

The chapters on the history of GME, credentialing, funding and manpower are primarily informational; the remainder are largely the product of personal experience and that of other colleagues in the field of medical education.

Among the major challenges to contemporary medicine are issues relating to credentialing, teaching and learning, performance assessment, professionalism, technologic innovation, research training, the supply and distribution of physicians, and funding, all of which bear directly on GME.

Realizing that I have done full justice to none of these topics – and my debt to many for what I have done – it is my hope that these reflections will stimulate concerned individuals, organizations, and the research needed for continued improvement in what and how we teach residents.

Frank C. Wilson
August 2009

About the Author

Frank Wilson was born in Rome, Georgia and graduated from the Darlington School, Vanderbilt University, and the Medical College of Georgia. He was a resident and fellow in Orthopaedics at Columbia-Presbyterian Medical Center in New York City, after which he joined the faculty at the University of North Carolina School of Medicine, where he served as Chief and Director of the Residency Program in Orthopaedics, Director of the Musculoskeletal Curriculum, and Instructor in the UNC undergraduate Honors Program, teaching literature courses on Thomas Wolfe and great books of the Western world.

Professional recognitions include designation as a Markle Scholar in Academic Medicine, the Nicholas Andry Award for Orthopaedic Research, Alpha Omega Alpha, and his selection to the leadership positions in the Association of Orthopaedic Chairmen, Council of Academic Societies (AAMC), American Orthopaedic Association, Residency Review Committee for Orthopaedics (ACGME), American Board of Orthopaedic Surgery, and Thomas Wolfe Society. He has been honored by the University of North Carolina with a Kenan Professorship and the Thomas Jefferson Award, and by the American Orthopaedic Association with its Distinguished Clinician–Educator Award.

Dr. Wilson has authored or co-authored over 165 publications (30 on education), five books (four on education), a play, and a collection of essays on the relationship between medicine and the humanities. He has taught more than 6000 students and overseen the education of over 100 residents.

Acknowledgments

For whatever insight, direction, and impetus for change achieved in this work, I owe much to many: to Dr. David C. Leach for his abiding support and gracious Foreword; to my ever able and willing wife Ann, who repeatedly strengthened my tenuous connection to the electronic world; to Nancy J. Rohr for her skill and patience in preparation of the manuscript; to the staffs of the AAMC and ACGME for providing essential data and suggestions; to Drs. Colin G. Thomas, F. Alden Dunham, and Shepard R. Hurwitz for their encouragement and advice; to Catherine Wells for her persistence with permissions, and to Donald B. Kettlekamp, whose unfailing answer to the difficulties I expressed in completing this book was "Remember, you don't have to do this." He was, of course, right.

1

Graduate Medical Education

Then and Now*

By way of overview, this survey begins with a historical fantasy and ends with a prophecy, but it deals most of all with an evolving present.

It is probably presumptuous for a specialist to address generic issues in graduate medical education (GME) because of the biases inherent in greater familiarity with one's own specialty; and even deeper contrition is felt for the many numerical data points, which are intended to suggest direction and trend rather than factual finality.

HISTORY

The American system of graduate medical education was born at the Johns Hopkins Hospital in the late 1800s. While records of its conception are sketchy, one might imagine a scenario in which Dr. Henry Hurd, the first director of the hospital, called William Welch, Dean of the inchoate School of Medicine, and Drs. Osler, Halsted, and Kelly to his office to discuss hospital operations and to express his displeasure at being the only physician on call the previous night to take care of all emergencies. In spite of Welch's

---

* Published in part in "The accreditation of graduate educational programs in orthopedic surgery" *Clinical Orthopaedics and Related Research*. 1990; **257**: 18–21. It appears here with the permission of Lippincott Williams and Wilkins.

compelling explanation that they had been planning the formation of the medical school, this experience convinced Dr. Hurd that a system of supplemental coverage was needed for the full-time staff. Osler concurred, noting that the responsibility for working up every patient in the hospital precluded the scholarly activity central to the mission of the faculty. Dr. Welch pointed out that they could not rely on part-time faculty, since they were more concerned with making money and, as such, were not good role models for students. He suggested that the hospital offer an apprenticeship to bridge the gap from medical school to practice. Halsted concurred with the need for help with routine aspects of patient care but pointed out that with departmental funds already under severe pressure, there was no source of payment for these positions. Hurd suggested that they be given room, board, and uniform in lieu of cash. Osler agreed, noting that the learning opportunities for these young men would be compensation enough.

And so it remained for almost 60 years, without, it should be added, the suggested indifference to the experience obtained by the house staff.

Thus, graduate medical education grew up in the hospital, as opposed to undergraduate education, which was a product of the medical school environment. These young physicians were called residents, a word derived from an era when they resided, or were "interned," in the hospital on essentially a full-time basis.[1]

GROWTH

Most of the growth of GME occurred after World War II: in 1940 there were about 5000 residents; in 2008, almost 110 000 were on duty in 8595 programs, over half of which were subspecialty programs. Of the 127 accredited disciplines in which a medical graduate might specialize, 26 were "primary" specialties and the remainder subspecialties in a primary discipline.[2] In 2007, 42% of all residents were in the primary programs of Internal Medicine, Family Practice, Pediatrics or Obstetrics-Gynecology.[3] Approximately 21% of all residents matching into PG-1 programs in recent years have been international medical graduates (IMGs).[4]

EDUCATIONAL GOALS AND INCENTIVES

The goals of GME are to prepare physicians for the practice of medicine, continued professional development, and lifelong learning.

For the physician, there are a number of incentives for graduate training. Completion of a residency, although not required for practice, leads to enhanced clinical skills. Certification or eligibility for certification by a specialty board is required for admitting privileges in most hospitals, and professional fees are often higher for specialists than for generalists who perform the same service.

CURRICULA

There are few formal curricula for GME; however, the content of the educational experience is specified in general terms for each discipline by its specialty board and residency review committee (RRC). Many requirements are common to the educational programs of all specialties, although the emphasis varies from discipline to discipline.

The time needed for competence in a discipline is determined by its specialty board; the range is from two to six years of graduate education.

INFLUENCES

In addition to evolving knowledge and technology, factors that influence GME are academic medical centers (AMCs), credentialing bodies, class size and composition, student specialty preferences, methods of health care delivery, economic constraints, and governmental regulations.

The AMC bears upon GME in a variety of ways. The program director is responsible for establishing the educational goals of the program, the selection, supervision, and evaluation of residents, counseling, censure and dismissal of residents whose performance is unsatisfactory, provision of adequate facilities and teaching staff, resident stress and working conditions, and communications with the residency review committee. With increasing fiscal constraints and emphasis on institutional responsibility, the hospital director has played a larger role in these determinations. By their number of graduates, medical schools affect the supply of residency positions. Also, deans and faculties of medicine have come to recognize more formally the importance of residents in the education of medical students.

The role of credentialing bodies is discussed in the following chapter.

Class size also affects GME. In 1967, there were 7743 graduates of U.S. medical schools; a number that had more than doubled by 2007, although in the last 25 years the annual number of graduates has not changed appreciably (15 802 to 16 139).[5] Between, 1967 and 2007, the number of accredited U.S. medical schools increased from 84 to 126 – a growth rate of 33% in 40 years.[6] Three additional schools were established in 2008. The average first-year class size in 1967 was 107; in 2006 it was 139, with enrollments ranging from 43 to 299.[7]

Because there is no centralized control over medical education, decisions about class size, which have national implications in the aggregate, are made institutionally, often because of factors of intense but localized significance, such as dependence on state subsidies and unmet needs for physician services in the community.

In 2006, the Association of American Medical Colleges (AAMC) Center for Workforce Studies, anticipating a physician deficit in the U.S. over the next several decades, called for medical schools approved by the Liaison Committee on Medical Education to increase their enrollment by 30% over 2002 levels during the next decade. Fully implemented, this change would increase medical school enrollments by almost 5000 per year.[8] If the number of IMGs in GME programs remains constant, the total number of residency positions will have to be increased to accommodate them, which would require removal of current Medicare restrictions on GME funding.

Changes in the gender mix of medical school classes have also influenced the graduate arena. Women constituted 11% of first year medical school classes in 1970; by 2007 this number had risen to 48%. Over 70% of all residents in Pediatrics and Obstetrics-Gynecology in 2007 were women.[9]

The ratio of minority students has also risen steadily. Black Americans made up 6.7% of medical school graduates in 2007, up from 5.1% in 1978, while the Asian population in GME increased from 2.6% to 20.4% over the same period.[10]

Student preferences have also affected GME in recent years. The percentage of students entering the primary care disciplines dropped from 49 to 44 between 2002 and 2007, and the percentage of primary care residents who pursued subspecialty training has risen steadily, reaching 58% in Internal Medicine and 33% in Pediatrics in 2007.[11,12]

The extent to which specialty choices have been influenced by indebtedness is problematic; however, in 2007, 65% of medical graduates had debts of over $100 000, up from 13% in 1997.[13]

Changes in health care delivery have had a major impact on residency training. Fueled by mounting costs, the system of health care delivery has changed at a revolutionary rather than an evolutionary rate. Studies and operations previously performed during hospitalization now are done on an outpatient basis, and hospital recuperation periods have been shortened by discharging patients as soon as "clinically appropriate." As a result, patients in the hospital have more acute and complex problems that require greater intensity of care. These changes have altered the nature of residency training by confining resident experience to sicker patients, often with esoteric disorders rarely encountered by physicians in practice. Nor does the resident have the opportunity to participate in many critical aspects of patient care that take place before and after admission. Surgical education in particular has become more limited to the operating room, which, coupled with less patient contact pre- and postoperatively, has concentrated resident education on technology rather than comprehensive surgical care.

Because of this shift in the provision of health care from hospital to nonhospital sites, physicians-in-training are spending more time in remote clinics and operatories, with no opportunities in the latter for pre- or postoperative contact with the patient. Many hospitals have increased ambulatory care experiences for their house officers, but differing educational philosophies and numerous operational and funding problems confront program directors who make greater use of ambulatory settings for education.

Economic constraints have also exerted pressures on graduate education. Teaching hospitals incur significant added costs in providing GME programs. While third-party payers initially paid teaching hospitals for both patient care and education, these policies have changed. In the Consolidated Omnibus Budget Reconciliation Act (COBRA) of 1985, limits were imposed on Medicare's open-ended responsibility to pay medical education costs. As a result, Medicare payments fail to cover Medicare's share of hospital costs for medical education – and voices in Congress have questioned whether *any* educational costs should be paid.

Payment practices by private health insurers have changed as hospitals entered into fixed-price contracts with organized health care systems. Since the payer's objective is to purchase care at the lowest possible cost, they are reluctant to pay extra for residency education.

Whatever the level, length, and method of funding, it seems appropriate for those who utilize resident services, namely the sick, to bear the service component of resident costs; and for all of society to share the educational costs, as everyone benefits from well-trained physicians. The problem lies in teasing apart service and education, since learning occurs during the provision of service.

Legislative constraints upon the admission of IMGs to graduate programs in the U.S. have waxed and waned. Until 1975, IMGs were welcomed under an open-door policy based upon a perceived need for more physicians. As shortage gave way to imminent surplus, Congress, in the mid-1970s, amended the Immigration and Nationality Act that made it more difficult for alien (vs. U.S. citizen) graduates of foreign medical schools to practice here. Even so, from 1990 to 2007, alien foreign graduate applicants to U.S. residency programs increased from 17% to 31% of the total.[14] Unfortunately, the Liaison Committee on Medical Education (LCME) is limited in scope to medical schools in the U.S. or Canada, which raises questions about the quality of foreign medical schools that have no comparable accreditation process.

Historically, medicine has been a self-regulating vocation; however, both federal and state governments have taken increased oversight and regulatory interests in medicine and medical education. COBRA included a provision mandating the establishment of a Council on Graduate Medical Education (COGME). This Council has issued informational reports to Congress and the Secretary of Health and Human Services almost annually since 1988 on a wide variety of topics, including the supply and distribution of physicians, financing of GME, women and minority groups in medicine, IMGs, the education of physicians, and managed care.

ISSUES AND OPTIONS

It is easier to see where GME has been and is than where it is going. The only thing certain about the future is its uncertainty. Changes will be proposed, and medical leaders and organizations must decide which of these are needed, which are tolerable, and which are unacceptable. Those aspects of GME that should be protected include:

1 The preservation of educational primacy
   With sicker patients and lower per patient levels of funding, clinical pressures on residents will continue to increase, eroding the time available for teaching, study, and research. To preserve this time, it may become necessary for academic medical centers to define that proportion of resident activity dedicated to educational pursuits, pay for it from a separate pocket, and ensure its occurrence.

2 Control of the educational process by educators
   It is unlikely that bureaucrats will make sounder educational decisions than educators; however, to the extent that educators fail to recognize the social, economic, and ethical – as well as the medical – dimensions of residency training, we may expect the control of medical education to pass from the hands of educators to those of lawmakers.

3 Adequate supervision
   Residents should be supervised in all phases of the educational process, for most of which on-site faculty are necessary.

Inadequate supervision may be responsible for more errors in patient care than resident fatigue.[15]

4 Continuity of care

This essential has received too little emphasis, but understanding fully the context of a patient in which a disease or disorder occurs is critical to the appropriate management of that disorder. Surgical results, for example, are often as deeply rooted in the expectations and needs of a patient as they are in the pathology of his or her disease; and when rehabilitation is necessary for a patient to realize the full benefits of a therapeutic intervention, the responsible physician should remain involved in the planning and direction of the rehabilitation program. Physicians should maintain their logical role as leaders of the health care team.

5 Stable funding

Given the approaching crisis in Medicare funding and the need to increase the number of physicians (and hence residents) in the U.S., other funding sources must be found. With the clinical productivity of faculty members restricted by supervisory and teaching responsibilities, it is unrealistic to expect funding from academic practice plans to support resident education.

6 Educational breadth

The lack of educational breadth seen among many specialists represents primarily a deficiency in baccalaureate education; however, formal instruction in such topics as professionalism, interactive skills, biostatistics, medicine and the law, medical economics, and medical information and practice systems, must find their way into graduate education. An institutionally sponsored core curriculum for these subjects would increase the comprehensiveness and quality of individual disciplinary offerings in a time-effective manner. Maintaining educational breadth will become increasingly important to avoid the tunnel vision engendered by increasingly specialized knowledge and technology.

7 Finally, we must hold our residents to high standards Residents who are unable, unwilling, or unscrupulous become practitioners with the same traits. We monitor cognition and motor skills well, but must improve our capacity to assess attitudes and values, since these qualities regulate the expression of innate abilities and skills – acknowledging that because of their subjective nature, they will never be precisely quantifiable.

It is upon these grounds that the battle for GME must be fought and won if medicine is to remain a highly esteemed profession. To the extent that its practitioners couple competence with dedication to the welfare of their patients and society, health care will benefit.

REFERENCES

1 Wilson FC. Graduate medical education: prescriptions for change. *Report of the Board of Directors' Workshop on Education*. Williamsburg, VA: American Academy of Orthopaedic Surgeons; 1985. pp. 15–30.

2 Accreditation Council for Graduate Medical Education Data Base. Chicago, IL; 2008–09.

3 *Graduate Medical Education Data Resource Book*. Chicago, IL: Accreditation Council for Graduate Medical Education; 2006–07. pp. 30–2.

4 *AAMC Data Book*. Washington, DC: Association of American Medical Colleges; 2008. p. 69.

5 Ibid. pp. 9–10.

6 Ibid. p. 5.

7 Barzansky B, Etzel SI. Medical Schools in the United States, 2006–07. *JAMA*. 2007; **298**(9): 1071–7.

8 *AAMC Statement on the Physician Workforce*. Washington, DC: Association of American Medical Colleges; 2006.

9 *AAMC Data Book*, op. cit. pp. 28–9, 80–1.

10 *AAMC Data Book*, op. cit. pp. 25–7.

11 *Graduate Medical Education Data Resource Book*, op. cit. pp. 88–90.

12 Brotherton SE, Etzel SI. Graduate Medical Education, 2006–07. *JAMA*. 2007; **298**(9): 1081–7.
13 *AAMC Data Book*, op. cit. p. 58.
14 Ibid. p. 69.
15 Fletcher KE, David SQ, Underwood W, *et al*. Systematic review: effects of resident work hours on patient safety. *Ann Intern Med*. 2004; **141**: 851–7.

2

Credentialing in Medicine

Protecting the Public*

In this chapter, "credentialing" is used as an umbrella term for the accreditation of programs and the licensure and certification of individual practitioners.

Physicians recognize credentialing as one of the rites of passage in medical education; less well understood is the importance of credentialing to the public, namely, that self-developed and enforced standards of learning are one of the pillars of accountability upon which a profession rests.

ACCREDITATION[1,2]

The accreditation of graduate medical education (GME) began in 1914 when the American Medical Association (AMA) published a list of hospitals approved for internships. During the ensuing decades, the American Board of Medical Specialties (ABMS), the American Hospital Association (AHA), the Association of American Medical Colleges (AAMC), and the Council of Medical Specialty Societies (CMSS) joined the AMA to form what since 1981 has been known as the Accreditation Council for Graduate Medical Education

---

* Parts of this chapter were published in "Credentialing in medicine" *The Annals of Thoracic Surgery*. 1993; **55**: 1345–8. They appear here with the permission of that Journal.

(ACGME). Each of these five member organizations appoints four representatives to the Council.

The ACGME carries out its accreditation mission by establishing Institutional Requirements for graduate medical education, and by developing procedures to accomplish the accreditation process. The Council delegates much of its work to Residency Review Committees (RRCs), which are composed of volunteer physicians in 26 primary specialty areas. The RRCs, in addition to writing the Program Requirements for residency training in their areas, make accreditation decisions about programs in that discipline.

Each RRC is sponsored by two or three organizations, including the AMA (through its Council on Medical Education), the appropriate specialty board, and often a major specialty society.

The accreditation of residency programs is based upon their compliance with standards published by the ACGME. This publication is updated annually and contains the Institutional Requirements, the Common Program Requirements that apply to all residency programs, and the Program Requirements for each discipline. As of 2008, Program Requirements had been published for 127 disciplines, including subspecialty areas.

Institutional Requirements specify a hospital's obligations for the support of its GME programs. An institution must state in writing why it sponsors GME, and how its resources are distributed for educational purposes. The sponsor is also expected to provide an environment conducive to learning, assistance to program directors in carrying out their educational responsibilities, and assurance that residents are appropriately supervised, counseled, evaluated, and provided with due process. Institutional Requirements, almost ignored for years, are now stressed by the ACGME.

Residency accreditation. Although their emphasis varies among programs, Program Requirements usually include graduated clinical responsibility, in which faculty supervision is reduced with advancing abilities of the resident; continuity in patient care, which specifies that residents have ample opportunity to evaluate the effectiveness of therapeutic interventions; instruction in basic science, which includes formal instruction linked to clinical pathophysiology; and research experience, with requisite time, space, funding, and supervision. Faculty members are expected to serve as appropriate role models by producing and publishing their own research findings.

In 2001, the ACGME, seeking to bring a performance focus to the design and conduct of GME programs, adopted requirements for resident proficiency in six areas of competency; 1) patient care that is compassionate, appropriate, and effective for the treatment of health problems and the promotion of health; 2) interpersonal and communication skills that result in effective information exchange with patients, their families, and professional associates; 3) professionalism in carrying out occupational responsibilities, adherence to ethical principles, and sensitivity to a diverse patient population; 4) adequate medical knowledge of established and evolving biomedical, clinical, and cognate sciences, and the application of this knowledge to patient care; 5) use of practice-based learning to evaluate his/her practices, appraise and assimilate scientific evidence, and improve patient care; and 6) knowledge of systems-based practice by demonstrating an awareness of, and responsiveness to, the larger system of health care, and the ability to call on system resources for optimal care. Each of these areas is appropriate and necessary; however, faculties have traditionally emphasized patient care, interpersonal skills, and medical knowledge above other qualities, which suggests a need for weighting the competencies. It is also clear that evaluation can be made more effective by soliciting input from nurses, patients, and peers, in addition to that supplied by the faculty. Even so, valid and reproducible measurement of such behaviors and attitudes as professionalism, systems-based practice, and practice-based learning at the resident level remains problematic.

The minimum time for completion of GME in a specialty must be specified; however, this period may be extended for residents who do not reach the developmental milestones at the expected time.

The accreditation process takes place in either existing or new programs. Existing programs are reviewed in cycles of five years or less, as determined by the RRC. Program directors provide specific information about the clinical, educational, and research activities of the residents and faculty. A surveyor then visits the program and interviews faculty, residents and an institutional representative to assess the accuracy of this information. The program information and the surveyor's report are reviewed by the RRC, which then decides whether or not the program is in "substantial compliance" with the ACGME Requirements.

For a new program, the review begins when the program director applies formally to the executive director of the RRC. Program information is submitted by the program director to the RRC; if paper compliance exists, provisional accreditation is granted for a period not to exceed four years. After a survey, which allows a comprehensive review by the RRC, full accreditation is granted for substantial compliance.

In addition to the favorable actions of provisional and full accreditation, there are two major adverse rulings: *probationary*, given when programs are not in substantial compliance; and *withdrawal*, which may follow continued noncompliance of programs with provisional or probationary status.

Adverse decisions by the RRC may be appealed. The appeals process occurs in two phases. Phase I is a request by the program director for reconsideration by the RRC. If the RRC sustains its decision, the program may enter Phase II by appealing this judgment to the ACGME, at which time the decision is reviewed by a panel of physicians in the specialty appointed by the ACGME. By allowing the program director to respond to a potential adverse action before a final decision is made, it may become possible to eliminate phase I. Historically, about 50% of initially adverse RRC decisions are reversed.

Fellowship accreditation. Fellowship accreditation became a focused issue for the ACGME in the early 1980s because of mounting concern over the rapid and haphazard proliferation of postgraduate educational experiences. At that time, "fellowships" were usually initiated by an individual in specialty practice. The duration and timing of the fellowships, even in the same subspecialty, varied considerably; and neither content nor achievement levels were specified. Many fellowships included an investigative component, although the resulting publications were usually retrospective reviews that reflected scholarship rather than research. Finally, no minimal standards existed for the content or duration of the educational experience. Rather, upon completion of an arbitrary training period, the affiliated hospital awarded the trainee a certificate. In short, any additional piece of specialized training could be, and often was, called a fellowship.

Although a number of thoughtful physicians expressed concern over the fragmentation of medicine by subspecialization, the proliferation of fellowships continued, largely because of public demand and impetus from residents, fellowship directors, and, somewhat paradoxically, residency program directors. Fellowships are attractive to residents because they offer deeper knowledge, greater procedural skills, a more controllable lifestyle, a contained area for continued mastery, and the probability of a higher income. Fellowship directors are attracted by opportunities to disseminate their philosophy and techniques, expand their clinical coverage (and its associated charge base), increase their research productivity, and share the teaching load. For the residency program directors, a fellow is less costly than a faculty member and can do almost as much – often including billing for services (only by fellows in unaccredited programs) and taking night call. Finally, as more fellows come into the system and dilute the experience of residents, it becomes more necessary for residents to seek fellowships, which creates a type of "feedback" loop.

In 1981, responding to the lack of standards for fellowships, concerned organizations, including the ACGME, began to consider ways in which fellowships could be monitored for academic rigor. Aided by these discussions, the RRCs set about developing standards for fellowship education. It had become apparent that at least one year was needed to provide adequate clinical experience, although some believed that one year was too short. Achievement of the requisite academic dimensions, especially depth and diversity of faculty, seemed more likely if the fellowship program was associated with other academic programs where research facilities and personnel were already in place, which led to the requirement that fellowships be affiliated with an approved residency program, unless affiliation was precluded by geographic constraints.

Thus, important steps have been taken to protect the quality of fellowship and residency education; but we must continue to emphasize the principles upon which accreditation is based: autonomy, impartiality, expertise, accountability, and due process to justify the public trust that adequate standards have been met.

LICENSURE

Granting of licensure, the legal authority for medical practice, is the responsibility of individual states, most of which require graduation from an accredited medical school, passing an examination acceptable to their medical licensing board, and one year of GME.

The major responsibility for licensure examinations belonged for many years to the National Board of Medical Examiners (NBME), a private, voluntary, medical testing organization that was established in 1915 and offered a three-part examination covering basic sciences, clinical knowledge, and diagnostic and therapeutic problems.

An alternative to the NBME examination was developed in 1968 by the Federation of State Medical Boards (FSMB), which offered a single two-day examination called the Federal Licensing Examination (FLEX) that was accepted by all states.

Since 1992 there has been a single, uniform examination pathway to licensure for both U.S. graduates and IMGs, the United States Medical Licensing Examination, which is co-sponsored by the NBME and the FSMB. As with the earlier NBME examination, there are three steps: Step 1 assesses understanding and application of biomedical science; Step 2 examines knowledge and understanding of clinical science essential for supervised patient care; Step 3 evaluates medical knowledge for unsupervised practice.

CERTIFICATION[3]

The primary purpose of certification is to serve the best interests of the public. The benefits that accrue to the profession are the result of success in achieving that goal.

As the ACGME is the umbrella organization for the RRCs, the ABMS is the corresponding organization for the 24 specialty boards, but there is an important difference: the ACGME has veto power over actions of the RRCs, whereas the ABMS cannot veto actions of individual boards.

The ABMS was formed in 1933 as the Advisory Board of Medical Specialties by representatives from primary boards, the AMA Council on Medical Education, the AAMC, the AHA, the Federation of State Medical Licensing Boards, and the National Board of Medical Examiners. In 1970, the name was changed to the American Board of Medical Specialties (ABMS), which became a founding parent of the Liaison Committees on Undergraduate, Graduate, and Continuing Medical Education.

The primary function of the ABMS is to assist its member boards in their efforts to certify and maintain the competence of specialists. It may coordinate, lead, or participate in collective efforts to these ends. As desired by member boards, the ABMS may also represent them in relationships with other organizations and provide information to the public, the government, the profession, and, especially, to its members. Underlying each of these functions is a commitment to the health of the public through activities that strengthen the qualifications of a physician for practice.

It is also important to understand the roles of other related groups: individual specialty boards function to certify candidates who possess the knowledge and skills necessary to meet established educational standards; academic groups provide leadership in specialty medicine through education and research; and specialty societies determine the dimensions of the specialty. Thus, the boards that judge, the faculty groups that lead, and the specialty societies that legislate may be likened to the judicial, executive, and legislative branches of the government. Each of these arms provides balances and checks to the privileges of the others. This separation of duties is critical, since no one body can credibly lead, legislate, and judge.

The first board to incorporate was the American Board of Ophthalmology, formed in 1917. Since then, 23 additional boards have been recognized by the ABMS. So rigorous are standards for recognition of a new board that only six new boards have been approved in the past 50 years, and none since 1996. About 85% of all U.S. physicians are certified specialists.

Subspecialty certification. The recognition of special qualifications for subspecialty certification began in the 1940s when seven subspecialty boards were incorporated into the American Board of Internal Medicine. In 1973, the ABMS Bylaws were revised to provide policy guidelines and procedures for the certification of Special Competence. To qualify, a subspecialty was, and is, required to demonstrate: 1) a distinct body of scientific knowledge; 2) a sizable group of physicians who concentrated their practice in the subspecialty; 3) the support of national professional societies; 4) educational programs of appropriate length and complexity (usually one to three years) that could not be included in the residency; and 5) candidates that were certified in the basic specialty before taking an examination in the subspecialty.

The subcertification process must be initiated by a specialty society, with the advice and consent of the specialty board.

While early subspecialization led to certificates of *special* qualifications, the ABMS decided in 1984, three years later, also to issue certificates of *added* qualifications, which were modifications of the primary certificate rather than separate certificates. A second difference was that boards could accept for special certification applicants other than their own diplomates who met the requirements for such certification, whereas added qualifications were issued only to applicants from the issuing board. The confusion engendered by these subtle differences has led the ABMS to recommend a single term, "Subspecialty Certification in . . ." to designate all subspecialty qualifications.[4] It is also noteworthy that no subspecialty certificates are offered simply to encompass isolated technical or procedural skills.

While the number of specialty boards has grown slowly, subspecialty proliferation has occurred at a rapid rate. As of 2008, there were 113 subspecialties recognized by the ABMS, with more undoubtedly to follow.

Traditionally, program accreditation by the ACGME was authorized only after certification in the subspecialty had been approved by the ABMS. That practice changed in 1984 when the ACGME authorized accreditation of orthopaedic fellowships for which no certificates were in place. They took that step to ensure the quality of fellowship programs at a time when subcertification was a political anathema within that specialty. The ripples from that decision led in 1989 to an ABMS/ACGME conference on accreditation without certification. Consensus recommendations from that meeting included: 1) recognition that both accreditation and certification are necessary; 2) accreditation could occur without certification; but 3) the need for certification of such groups would have to be reviewed at least every five years – which might result in the perception of either a diminishing need for accreditation or a need for certification.

Although definitive recommendations were not forthcoming from this conference, it raised critical issues of flexibility and the need for independence of certification and accreditation, which helped in meeting the complex credentialing challenges posed by the emergence of new areas of subspecialty practice.

MAINTENANCE OF CERTIFICATION

Passing an examination after a residency does not confer competence in perpetuity. Basic information must be retained and used, obsolete information discarded, and new knowledge acquired to maintain a high standard of practice; therefore, periodic reassessment is rational and necessary. The problem is not with the concept but with the method. The certification process emphasizes cognitive competence – what a physician knows – for which an examination is appropriate. For Maintenance of Certification (MOC), the principal concern is performance in practice – what a physician does – which, because it reflects attitudes and skills as well as erudition, is more complex and difficult to quantify. Performance is similar to an iceberg: the small, visible top, like knowledge, may be clearly defined and reliably measured; but the greater, submerged part, composed of those qualities that determine how one's knowledge is used, is dimly perceived and defies precise definition. Thus, an ongoing challenge for all specialty boards is how to measure performance reliably for MOC.

Discussions of the need and means for assessing continuing competence have a long history. In 1940, the ABMS Commission on Graduate Medical Education stated, "As the certifying boards become established . . . they may find it desirable to use certificates that are valid for a stated period." In 1973, a resolution stated "that the ABMS adopts in principle and urges concurrence . . . with the policy that voluntary recertification . . . become an integral part of all certification." The first two boards to adopt that policy were the American Board of Family Practice and the American Board of Internal Medicine (ABIM). The ABIM administered its first recertification examination in 1974 as a voluntary process; however, because only a small percentage of certified internists took the examination, they decided, beginning in 1990, to implement time-limited certification. By 2006, all 24 primary boards were issuing only time-limited certificates, which are valid for 6–10 years.

Most objections to MOC have come from practitioners, whose major concern is the content of the evaluation, since many professionals have limited their area and style of practice. Other concerns relate to expense, disputes about the ability to measure the performance of a physician in practice, and, although unspoken, fear of failure, with its economic implications.

These concerns led to exploration of a number of avenues for MOC, most of which included a combination of cognitive assessment, peer review, and continuing medical education.

Successful completion of MOC requirements should signify that anyone originally awarded a certificate possesses and *utilizes*, 6–10 years later, competencies at least equal to those possessed on the day the certificate was issued. Following the adoption by the ABMS of the six core competencies for resident evaluation, the ABMS developed a program for the assessment of MOC that consisted of four components: professional standing, a commitment to lifelong learning with periodic self-assessment, cognitive expertise, and evaluation of performance in practice.

Optional implementation of MOC will require further study of: 1) means for valid and reliable assessment of the possession and use of requisite knowledge, skills, and attitudes; 2) ways to deal with the heterogeneity of practice within certain disciplines; 3) legal defensibility; and 4) cost. All boards must be in compliance by 2010. As electronic data collection and transfer become routine, reportable data could be collected from hospitals and offices and sent to specialty boards for consideration as performance measures for MOC.

Whatever the method, periodic efforts to eliminate, modify, or control the MOC process have occurred by those at risk; however, since credentialing has, as its primary purpose, protection of the public, it is plain that standards of performance must be set and implemented without the friendly persuasion of those to whom they apply. While boards cannot and should not operate in a vacuum, the perception of autonomy is crucial to the credibility of any credentialing process; in fact, to the degree that conflict between public and personal interest is answered in favor of the public, credentialing bodies achieve nobility of purpose.

ISSUES AND OPTIONS

Quality in education, like quality in research and patient care, requires time for reflection, preparation, assessment, and adjustment in addition to the activity itself. The expansion of clinical effort driven by managed care has reduced the time needed to protect these aspects of quality. Quantity, beyond a certain critical mass, undermines quality. The expected increase in numbers of medical students and residents will in itself extend the time required for performance evaluation, as will the increasing complexity of the accreditation and certification processes. At some point – sooner rather than later – simplification of credentialing processes must become a prominent consideration in decision-making.

Fortunately, the demand for quality assurance and accountability has been met, at least in part, by the expanded use of information technology to support electronic medical records and computerized order entry, which facilitates collection and transfer of performance data on physicians and hospitals to accrediting and certifying bodies.[5]

As in the past, major responsibilities for quality control will reside with accrediting and certifying bodies, but a team and systems approach in institutions, departments, and among health care workers is also needed to support a culture of quality in the rush to quantity. Critical to this end is the quality of resident education, which is linked closely to the level of patient care. Until resident education is expanded from a patient-specific approach to a systems-based perspective that includes other disciplines and health care professionals, the rules governing payment and accreditation, preventive medicine, and broad patterns of health care delivery, progress in quality improvement will be limited.

Accreditation, licensing, and certification will never be perfect processes, but that should not prevent the quest for better ones. Credentialing is a powerful tool that must not become so politically, emotionally, or bureaucratically entangled that it fails to serve the best interests of patients. If medicine abdicates its responsibility to impose credible standards on itself, our place will be taken by very interested but less knowledgeable others. Participants in the credentialing movement may take great pride in what has been accomplished. To build on this record of achievement, medicine must rededicate itself to the requirement of reasonable standards as a professional obligation, and to a continuing search for the most efficient means to meet those standards.

REFERENCES

1 Accreditation Council for Graduate Medical Education Data Base. Chicago, IL; 2008–09.

2 *Graduate Medical Education Data Resource Book.* Chicago, IL: Accreditation Council for Graduate Medical Education; 2006–07.

3 *American Board of Medical Specialties Annual Report and Reference Handbook.* Evanston, IL: American Board of Medical Specialties Research and Education Foundation; 2008.

4 DeRosa GP. *The American Board of Orthopaedic Surgery: a 75-year history.* Chapel Hill, NC: American Board of Orthopaedic Surgery; 2009.

5 Benjamin EM. Improving quality and safety at an academic health center. *Prescriptions for Excellence in Health Care*. Jefferson Medical College and Eli Lilly and Co. 2007; **2**: 7–9.

3

Teaching and Learning
Establishing an Educational Continuum

It has been said that there are three attributes that every man believes himself to possess: his ability to drive an automobile, his seductive powers, and his ability to teach. Highway accident statistics and the studies of Masters and Johnson suggest the improbability of the first two, and one has only to read the comments made by students in response to our educational efforts to wonder if they too are not suspect.

Ratings, however, are less a product of curriculum than of the enthusiasm, ability, and commitment of the teacher. Curriculum is not a substitute for personal involvement in the educational process, nor does it provide a destination for the educational experience. Curriculum is only one tool for getting there, and, like any tool, it should be used where it can exert the greatest effect. So the goal – where one wants to go with a curriculum – must be established first.

It is probably not far off the mark to suggest that the goal of medical education is the production of physicians who blend scientific knowledge and methodology with appropriate human values and skills in the practice of medicine. The scientific method – developing and testing a hypothesis – is difficult to teach, but it provides the means by which information and data may be evaluated and accepted or rejected. It is, in a sense, the discipline that a mind possesses, which is more important than any factual furnishings it has. Critical thinking is the centerpiece; information can be found in a book or on a web page. Though innate to experimental work, analytic thought is not confined to the research arena. Clinicians too must understand the essentiality of asking the right questions, proposing hypothetical answers, and collecting the data necessary to validate (or invalidate) their practices. They need to know which conclusions can be legitimately drawn from a given database, and which are inappropriate. To do so, they must be able to apply the principles of validity and reliability to the analysis of data.

Although learning goals for the cognitive domain have been established for each discipline by accreditation and certification requirements, there have been relatively few efforts to develop specific objectives for each phase of the educational continuum and to linking the instructional offerings in one phase with those in the next.

To address the discontinuities in musculoskeletal education, the orthopaedic faculty developed a curricular continuum for musculoskeletal education at the University of North Carolina School of Medicine in Chapel Hill.

Before graduate curricular planning could be done, certain assumptions had to be made about the educational experiences that had preceded it; therefore we developed educational objectives for each of the contact periods between Orthopaedics and the medical students, which included a two-week musculoskeletal course during the second year, a three-week clerkship (for 40% of the students) during the third year, and six one-month electives (taken by about 15% of the class) during the fourth year. The objectives for these courses focused on that material judged to be important for the practice of medicine by non-orthopaedic physicians. There was no intent or effort to make an orthopaedist out of every medical student.

Next, a basic surgical education program was developed for the first graduate year, the aim of which was to assist the prospective surgeon acquire the knowledge, skills, and attitudes necessary to ensure competence in those elements of surgery common to all surgical specialties. This curriculum encompassed 17 general headings or units, ranging from basic wound healing to the psychological aspects of surgery, from neonatology to gerontology. Each unit included an overall goal and specific educational objectives in the cognitive, psychomotor, and affective domains to achieve that goal. These objectives followed a year of weekly meetings by a committee representing most of the surgical disciplines – sessions that were often characterized by divergent opinions as to what constituted surgical commonalities. After accord was reached, the entire surgical faculty was invited to review and comment on the objectives, and many of their suggestions were incorporated into the final document.

Responsibility for the educational experience in each subject was assigned to a faculty member in the Department of Surgery – the unit director – who possessed particular expertise or interest in that area; and a period was set aside for basic surgical education, usually a Saturday morning seminar, for which an advance reading list had been distributed. This time was inviolate from all interruptions except emergencies. Basic psychomotor skills were formally covered in the animal laboratories, each surgical discipline being responsible for one session.

All first year surgical residents participated. Pre- and post-testing examinations were prepared by an examination committee from questions based on the educational objectives submitted by each unit director. Residents' scores improved each year by an average of 34% (range: 30–39%). Because it was impossible to determine how much of this gain resulted from basic surgical education and how much from informal, day-to-day clinical teaching, testing was discontinued after five years.

We did not establish a pass-fail level for the basic surgical educational course nor require remediation for areas of documented deficiency, although each resident's scores were made known to him or her for self-remediation.

Knowledge of house officers' prior education provided a firm base for the orthopaedic residency curriculum, which was divided into four parts: trauma, adult reconstructive orthopaedics, pediatric orthopaedics, and basic science. One faculty member wrote cognitive, psychomotor, and affective objectives for each section, after which these objectives were reviewed by the faculty, discussed, and rewritten until consensus was reached. There were again heated but honest disagreements as to what constituted core education, especially in psychomotor skills; but just when it seemed as though everything might go up in smoke, a compromise was reached that allowed the process to continue.

The development of surgical core curricula seemed appropriate and timely for a number of reasons: First, there were skills, attitudes and knowledge that should be possessed by surgeons that had not been clearly defined. Second, with increasing opportunities for students to enter specialized areas of surgery directly, there was a growing tendency to bypass many of the surgical commonalties. Third, as institutions assumed more responsibility for the integration and evaluation of their residency programs, specialty-specific curricula were needed to assure the education of competent specialists. Fourth, a clear statement of educational objectives was important to facilitate monitoring and evaluating the achievement and progress of house officers. Finally, these objectives could provide a basis for the design of subspecialty and continuing medical educational curricula.

Insofar as possible, the objectives were stated in behavioral terms. As Mager described, what the learner was expected to be able to do upon completion of the educational experience was determined, the conditions under which the learning experience would occur were stated, and an acceptable level of achievement was defined.[1]

The next, and very pertinent, question was, "So what?" Now that we had a curriculum, what were we going to do with it? We used it in the following way: a copy of the objectives was given to all residents when they started the program so that they could cover or review, at their own pace, the essentials of orthopaedic education. We also used the objectives to plan the structured portions of the educational program, such as clinical conferences, seminars, and basic science sessions.

Most subjects were covered in a lecture series spread over four years; the more common or complex topics were offered twice, and a few were left for unstructured educational experiences.

The third part of the cybernetic cycle, evaluation, followed. By knowing what had (and had not) been accomplished, subsequent educational experiences were adjusted appropriately. There were two criteria for acceptable performance in meeting the objectives of the curriculum: an average score for four years on the annual orthopaedic in-training examination at the 50th percentile or better; and, more importantly, faculty consensus – based on day-to-day observations throughout the residency – that the learner had acquired sufficient knowledge, technical and interpersonal skills, and attitudes, and had integrated them effectively in practice.

When possible, rotations were adjusted to provide greater exposure to areas of documented deficiency; however, throughout the program, primary responsibility for learning was laid at the feet of the residents: faculties teach, residents learn.

With annual curricular updates and one major revision, this program continued for 22 years. All residents who came through the program during this time passed the Orthopaedic Certifying Examination.

Certainly, educational objectives cannot cure all the ills that beset teaching programs; however, they provide a study guide for residents, a teaching outline for faculty, and a source of valid questions for examiners. They also facilitate communication among those responsible for the various phases of the educational continuum. Admittedly, the selection of objectives requires value judgments, especially in the affective and psychomotor domains, which might not be echoed in all institutions. However, were everyone to start as we did, from nothing, their educational value would probably not justify the time spent in their development. To the extent that our efforts guided other programs, less time in preparation may have made the use of educational objectives more feasible, contributing perhaps, in a better world, to national standards for education and assessment.

In emphasizing the *formal* curriculum, there is a caution not to overlook *informal* (social interaction and random contact) and *hidden* (behaviors rather than words) curricula, which are also critical determinants of professional behavior.

ISSUES AND OPTIONS

There are three essentials for learning in the clinical setting: 1) relevance – the learner's perception of a clear connection between the information offered and the solution of problems relevant to his or her career goals; 2) personal commitment by the learner (faculty teach; students learn); and 3) feedback – learners need to perceive clearly the gap between what they know and what they need to know, for which nonjudgmental feedback is critical; in fact, the teacher's time is often better spent in observation, assessment, and feedback than in delivering information.

In general, one acquires and retains information by using it to solve problems. Skills are mastered by repetition and practice; values and attitudes by association with those whom we respect and admire. The importance of role modeling for the latter – the hidden curriculum – cannot be overstated.

The search for ways to improve medical education should include a re-examination of the values underlying the profession. Values shape the world; they should hold pride of place in the intellectual community and drive the educational enterprise. Unfortunately the ethos that determined them in the past has been blurred by contravening trends of the present. Propelled by the explosive escalation of knowledge and technology, too little attention has been given to the humanistic values that should determine their use.

A sense of respect for this ideology begins with baccalaureate education. Too many college courses are taken simply to improve grade point averages or ease the passage to medical school, rather than to provide a base broad enough to accommodate both the *relevant* science and the obligations of medicine to society. With specialization, the educational pendulum has swung toward verticality in learning; however, early exposure to the liberal arts provides the broad horizontal base necessary to accommodate vertical growth. Though lacking the relevance and glamour of computer science, courses in philosophy, literature, history, and expository writing, along with courses in law and public policy, should be embedded in the premedical curriculum to enhance our sense of the world around us and to inculcate the accuracy, clarity, and brevity of expression needed to avoid the seemingly obligatory obfuscation of medical writing.

Philosophy introduces precepts of logic, ethics, and morality useful in every phase of medical practice. Literature, by exposing us to the insights and sensibilities of others, enables us to deepen our own. With understanding comes empathy.

A liberal education entails more than the accumulation of topical information; it should reinforce the interconnectedness of knowledge – humanistic, scientific, and technical. By studying mankind as well as his/her anatomy; by studying astronomy along with atoms and molecules, we develop a sense of proportion and balance, which informs later judgments. Content should be relevant and rigorous; equally critical is the way in which it is taught. Coherence is all; the best teachers enable us to see the forest by means of the trees.

In medical school, better advantage should be taken of the fourth year curriculum to prepare students for GME. Specialty societies should prepare a list of recommended rotations for students interested in that specialty, and faculty members in each discipline should be designated and available as mentors for students planning to pursue that specialty. Mentors could provide advice and assistance in scheduling fourth year electives, and assist students in preparing residency applications.

Given the inevitability of change, curricular offerings in GME should emphasize the importance of continuing education, adapting to new developments in science and practice, and forging firmer linkages between the phases of medical education.

Dreyfus has described the continuum of learning and skills acquisition as occurring in six stages: the *novice*, who learns by application of defined rules; the *advanced beginner*, who starts to apply the rules to new situations; the *competent learner*, who is able to vary the rules depending on context; the *proficient learner*, who applies skills and rules intuitively, distinguishing between critical and extraneous elements; and the *expert*, who can deal rapidly and accurately with complex situations, and who writes rather than reads the rules. The sixth stage, *master*, is distinguished by the response to surprise: experts hate surprises; masters welcome them. Ideally, this progression should occur seamlessly as medical students move from novice to advanced beginner, become competent and proficient as residents, and develop expertise with experience as practitioners, some of whom become masters.[2,3,4]

Using the Dreyfus model for skill development in medical practice, Carraccio, *et al.* have provided a list of appropriate behaviors for each stage in the development of physician competence, along with their implications for teaching and learning.[5]

Equally critical bridges are needed among clinical disciplines to provide comprehensive care for patients with multifaceted diseases. Bringing together multiple disciplines for the care of complex diseases benefits both the research and teaching of these disorders, as well as providing smoothly integrated, patient-centered care. Lateral integration among related disciplines, being easier to accomplish, occurs more frequently than vertical integration, which entails bringing together physicians from unrelated disciplines to manage a broader spectrum of disorders. Vertical integration in particular is beset with problems related to organization, management, scheduling conflicts, and flow of funds. Levin, *et al.* have suggested means of dealing with these issues to produce models of integrated care that are superior to stand-alone profit centers; however, the extent to which traditional departments will sacrifice the administrative and fiscal autonomy necessary to develop successful models of integrated care is uncertain.[6]

To improve residency training in the management of chronic disease, the AAMC established the Academic Chronic Care Collaborative in 2005, which has led to the formation in many institutions of interdisciplinary resident teams to care for patients with chronic, complex disorders.

While there is general agreement among medical educators on the importance of principles, the biologic bases for decision-making, and analytic thought, there is little consensus within individual specialties as to the optimal content or means for teaching it. Multiple variables – ability, commitment, student-faculty ratios, and means of assessment among them – obscure clear superiority for a particular curricular approach, whatever its theoretical benefits. National board scores have little comparative value because of the practice in some schools of teaching to the content of board examinations.

Critical to the success of any teaching program is the time and effort given by the faculty to its implementation. Teaching reduces time for patient care and research, both of which generate funds, which may explain the trend toward professors not professing. The teaching professor is further disadvantaged by promotion committees that find it difficult to assess either the quantity or the quality of instruction provided, and thus tend to shortchange its value in promotional decisions. Teaching, however, should be a responsibility of all faculty members, with the amount done by each determined by his or her interest and skill. Exceptional achievement should be recognized by promotion committees and a defined reimbursement structure.

It is a sad note in the history of medical education that faculty members have traditionally had so little preparation for their roles as teachers and mentors. Knowledge of subject was long considered preparation enough for teaching medicine; scant thought was given to curricular design, pedagogic techniques, learner evaluation, or educational research. Growing awareness of these issues has led to courses, programs, and fellowships to enhance the skills of clinician-educators.

Graffam, *et al.* studied clinicians' teaching practices to describe ideal teaching behaviors to establish a model for clinical instruction by which faculty could evaluate their own performance. Teaching practices were found to be made up of seven interrelated behaviors: engagement, conceptualization, discussion, modeling, measurement (and feedback), structure, and empowerment. Ideal behaviors were specified for each of these interrelated factors.[7]

A fellowship at Harvard, which includes a mentor and the requirement for an educational research study, is structured to occupy and compensate 20% of a fellow's time, thus enabling them to continue clinical responsibilities and departmental salaries with only schedule modifications.[8]

The program at McGill University, which is based on the Teaching Scholars Program at the University of North Carolina, has been operational since 1997. It includes two university courses, an educational research project, and educational workshops and seminars that emphasize educational leadership and scholarship. Scholars are expected to devote a minimum of one day a week for one year to complete the program. School-wide visibility of this program has increased the acceptance of excellence in teaching as a criterion for promotion.[9]

For teaching to assume its rightful place at the head of the academic table, there must be institutional values that recognize and reward teaching and innovation in education, honoring, as Jordan Cohen underscored, the "E" in GME.[10]

Finally, it should be emphasized that the context in which learning is expected to occur may be more important in fashioning the end product than any curriculum. It is critical to establish an atmosphere and environment in which scholarship is clearly practiced and valued, and rigorous intellectual discipline applied in both the investigative and clinical arenas. This emphasis should be apparent in conferences, on the wards, and in the operating room, as well as in the laboratory. It finds particular application in journal clubs, which should be approached as critical reading seminars that emphasize basic knowledge, analysis, methodology, and interpretation rather than as a series of informational summaries on clinical content. It is these qualities, blended with empathy and altruism, that we should be inculcating rather than trying to deliver all of the information needed for a lifetime of practice.

REFERENCES

1 Mager RF. *Preparing Instructional Objectives.* 3rd ed. Atlanta, GA: CEP Press Inc.; 1997.

2 Dreyfus SE, Dreyfus HL. A five-stage model of the mental activities involved in directed skill acquisition. Unpublished manuscript. Berkeley, CA: U.S. Air Force Office of Scientific Research, under contract F49620-79-0063 with the University of California, Berkeley; 1980.

3 Leach DC. Competence is a habit. *JAMA.* 2002; **287**: 243–4.

4 Dreyfus HL. *On the Internet.* London and New York, NY: Routledge; 2001. Ch. 3.

5 Carraccio CL, Benson BJ, Nixon LJ, *et al.* From the educational bench to the clinical bedside: translating the Dreyfus developmental model to the learning of clinical skills. *Acad Med.* 2008; **83**(8): 761–7.

6 Levin SA, Saxton JWF, Johns MME. Developing integrated clinical programs: it's what academic health centers should do better than anyone. So why don't they? *Acad Med.* 2008; **83**(1): 59–65.

7 Graffam B, Bowers L, Keene KN. Using observations of clinicians' teaching practices to build a model of clinical instruction. *Acad Med.* 2008; **83**(8): 768–74.

8 Hatem CJ, Lown BA, Newman LR. The academic health center coming of age: helping faculty become better teachers and agents of educational change. *Acad Med.* 2006; **81**(11): 941–4.

9 Steinert Y, McLeod PJ. From novice to informed educator: the teaching scholars program for educators in the health sciences. *Acad Med.* 2006; **81**(11): 969–74.

10 Cohen JJ. Honoring the "E" in GME. *Acad Med.* 1999; **74**(2): 108–13.

4

The Evaluation of Residents
Assessing Competent Performance

The stimulus for this topic was a statement by Henry Mankin that "All training chiefs are liars," which may explain why the assessment of house officers by their program director is of suspect value in the certification process.[1]

Dr. Mankin's observation raises the question of *why* program directors prevaricate when called upon to describe their products. If they were innately untruthful, they should lie as often about good as about bad residents – a phenomenon seldom observed. More likely explanations are that they are unwilling, unprincipled or unable. The unwilling program director gives evaluation a very low priority; the unprincipled director misrepresents to save face or avoid reprisal; the unable director is willing but unenlightened.

Effective residents differ little from specialty to specialty; all display efficient integration of the cognitive, affective, and motor domains. To this trinity of head, heart, and hands, we should add interpersonal skills, since they are of major importance and do not rest comfortably in another arena.

While there are unique difficulties with the evaluation of each domain, the affective area is the least amenable to objective evaluation because it requires assessment of the resident's personal attitudes and values – what he or she does when no one else is looking – including integrity, reliability, professionalism, dedication, humanism, stress tolerance, adaptability, and empathy.

Appraisal of the cognitive domain requires a search for the level of knowledge and the higher cognitive functions of comprehension, analysis, application and creation. Common sense is not included in this taxonomy, but it belongs. The contents of the cognitive domain have been defined in part by the educational requirements of each board, by certifying and in-training examinations, and by individual program directors. Unfortunately, very few disciplines have made more than token efforts to develop a formal curriculum for their specialty, which should precede and serve as a basis for testing rather than the reverse.

Evaluation of the motor domain requires assessment of the house officer's ability to perform specific motor movements, or patterns of movement in a coordinated and efficient manner, often under stressful conditions. Lippert and others have identified the specific motor skills necessary to perform complex clinical procedures as manual dexterity, three-dimensional perception, hand-eye coordination, and fine motor control.[2]

Interpersonal skills encompass those attributes necessary to leave a patient with a pleasant, satisfied feeling about an encounter. To produce an optimal outcome, however, such encounters usually entail input from all domains. For example, when a patient interaction extends through an operative procedure, a complex mix of affective and cognitive traits and skills occurs: the hands are the motor implements, but the selection, planning, and timing of the procedure are purely cognitive functions; obtaining the patient's trust and cooperation results largely from the interpersonal skills of the physician, and the entire encounter is driven by his or her attitudes and values.

With the content of evaluation in place, we are on firmer footing for the issues of "who," "how," "where," and "when."

The "who" should not be confined to the program director and faculty, since a house officer's performance in the presence of authority figures is less likely to depict what happens when no one who exercises control over his or her destiny is in the neighborhood. Written input should be obtained after each rotation from sources less threatening to the resident, including peers, nurses, patients, and perhaps the house officers themselves – a "360 degree" evaluation. Assessment of the affective domain entails judgment of behaviors against accepted standards. Another useful "how" is by critical incident studies, wherein specific behaviors that illustrate the presence or absence of a specific trait, attitude, or value are identified. The resident's performance is then examined for similar behavioral incidents to determine whether he or she demonstrates that trait.

The cognitive domain can be explored more objectively by the variety of written and oral examinations currently available, although techniques for assessment of higher cognitive functions need further development. An oral examination is often a better instrument for the appraisal of analytic abilities, logic, and thought processes – especially under stress, when a physician may have to make critical decisions. Program directors are less reliable for cognitive assessment than comprehensive written examinations, although a resident's ability to think on his or her feet and to create new knowledge may be better known to the program director.

Technical proficiency can be evaluated in motor skills laboratories with weighted checklists; however, the performance of an operation, with its associated cognitive and affective determinants, can, as yet, be judged only in the operating room by experienced surgeons – a setting in which standardization has been elusive.

The opportunities for direct observation of a house officer's performance must be taken where and when they occur: in the operating room, the emergency room, on the wards, in clinics, during conferences, and in the laboratory.

From these assessment methods, a composite rating can be formulated for discussion with the resident by the program director. When the feedback loop is closed in this manner, evaluation becomes formative as well as summative.

All six of the general core competencies (*see* Chapter 2 under Accreditation) embrace elements from multiple domains, though the elements vary somewhat in their importance from specialty to specialty.

After identifying the knowledge, attitudes, and skills needed in the core competencies and their means of assessment, their predictive validity can be established by tracking graduates through a practice period, comparing their performance (outcomes and complication rates) with ideal or community norms. Written and oral examinations and professional recognitions are more objective methods that can be used to make these judgments. Psychometrically valid and reliable instruments for measurement of the six competencies independently have not been found, in part because two of the competencies, systems-based practice and practice-based learning and improvement have been operationalized as properties of systems, not of individual trainees.[3] Therefore, it may be necessary to use the competencies to direct and coordinate more specific evaluations rather than attempting direct measurement of the individual competencies.

PSYCHOMETRIC CONSIDERATIONS

Competence signifies the capacity to function in a particular way or as having requisite or adequate ability. Defining competence helps assure the validity of certification procedures, since only after knowing what something is can one attempt to measure it. Also by spelling out the components of competence, planning of the educational experience is facilitated.

The term "competence" is often used interchangeably with "performance," but competence refers to ability, performance to what is actually done. One may know how to treat broken hips, be able to carry out appropriate operative management, and still not *do* it – thus performing inadequately while being completely competent. Performance thus relies more on affective or attitudinal qualities – commitment, empathy, and integrity – than competence.

Competence in a given area can be based on testing, consensus of expert judgments, and task analyses. It is not an all or nothing occurrence; rather, it is possessed in degrees, so that one is either more or less competent than a predetermined standard. The concept is made more complex in medicine by the existence of both horizontal and vertical dimensions. The horizontal dimensions are those of general medical competence, specialty competence, and competence in dealing with individual medical problems. Vertical dimensions are measured as minimal or maximal competence, or somewhere between, in each area.

General medical competence is, to some degree, assured by an MD degree, which includes such examinations as the U.S. Medical Licensing Examination or National Board examinations. Licensure examinations also measure general medical competence, as does the Visa Qualifying Examination. Specialty competence is determined by certifying board examinations and self-assessment techniques. Competence in dealing with individual patients may be assessed by practice audit and chart review.

Unfortunately, most proven testing devices deal primarily with the cognitive aspects of competence. Standardized techniques for evaluation of competence in psychomotor and interpersonal skills lag far behind.

For more reliable assessment of motor skills, surgical disciplines must further define the relationship between laboratory simulation and operating room performance – at least for purely motor activities. Weighted checklists, useful for the appraisal of motor skills in the laboratory, are less practical in the operating room. Wax and plaster carving and clay modeling may deserve further study, since they have been useful in identifying individuals with poor manual dexterity, hand-eye coordination, and three-dimensional perception.[4,5]

Interpersonal skills have been studied by a variety of techniques: 360 degree evaluations are useful, but simulated interviews have worked less well because of role-playing by both examiner and examinee. Conventional multiple choice questions, patient management problems, computerized simulation, videotapes of patient encounters and interaction analysis by direct observation with checklists have also been tried, but only interaction analysis has shown enough promise for objectifying physician performance to warrant further study.[6] If criteria for reliable scoring can be found, oral examinations may also afford an opportunity to assess interpersonal skills.

A major difficulty in rating interpersonal skills by any method is that diametrically opposite personality traits may be equally effective, depending upon the personality and attitudes of the patient.

The data upon which evaluation of affective traits can be based are less substantial, but this domain is critical since it regulates the expression of a person's abilities and skills. Because of their subjective nature, it is unlikely that attitudes and values will ever be as quantifiable as cognitive ability; however, because of its import, the affective domain deserves a particularly intensive research focus, beginning with the definition of its content elements, and critical incident studies to guide their evaluation.

Where objective evaluation is used, e.g. in multiple choice tests, the validity and reliability of the tests must be considered. Validity may be content, construct, or criterion-related. *Content* validity refers to the appropriateness of the test items for whatever is being measured. *Construct* validity pertains to how accurately test data reflect actual behavior. *Criterion-related* validity is said to be either concurrent (how well data from one test correlate with data from another) or predictive (the extent to which a test score predicts future performance). Reliability refers to the reproducibility of a test score over time or between observers. In general, a test is said to be reliable if it produces a Gaussian distribution of scores. The major determinant of reliability is the number of test items, but the quality of the examination and the number of individuals taking it are also important.

To determine validity, three essentials are necessary: a clear definition of competence, an appropriate test to measure it, and a pass-fail standard. The concurrence of all three is rare. Because most graduate disciplines lack well-defined, standardized curricula, their certifying board examinations have little content validity.

Another issue is whether testing should be criterion or norm-referenced. Traditionally, professional credentialing bodies have used a norm-referenced, or relative standard, examination, although this technique entails a percentage of failures, which may be undesirable, and it lacks validity in that the pass-fail standard is not related to the content of the examination; however, when course content has been defined, a level of mastery or pass-fail point can be set, although construct and predictive validities are difficult to determine. Criterion-referenced examinations also require that the most important content areas constitute a proportionately greater part of the examination; and the degree of "correctness" of a "wrong" answer should be (but rarely is) individually judged, since a given choice may be partially correct or totally incorrect.

Normative testing seeks a broad Gaussian distribution of grades. The value of each question may be assessed by the difficulty and discrimination indices. The difficulty index represents the proportion of students who answer a question correctly. Indices range from 0 to 1.00, with larger numbers representing an easier item and smaller numbers a harder one. The preferred range for the difficulty index is 0.20–0.80. Items outside of this range, especially those below 0.20, should be reviewed and possibly deleted. The discrimination index for a given item reports the difference in performance (for that item) of students whose overall test scores were high and those who had low scores. Discrimination indices range between 0.00 and 1.00 and can be negative. A negative index means that more low scorers on the entire test answered the question correctly than the higher scorers. When both the difficulty and discrimination indices are outside the normal range, questions should be deleted unless the item is well constructed, has no nonfunctioning or ambiguous distractors, and fairly represents content taught in the course.

ISSUES AND OPTIONS

It is often easier to do something than to know what one has done. Developing a curriculum is one thing; evaluating its effectiveness is more complex and difficult; however, as Dr. David Leach said, "Whatever we measure, we tend to improve."[7] By improving assessment, we improve learning, and by improving learning, we enhance patient care. Further, accurate assessment helps identify programmatic as well as individual educational deficits. Individual gaps suggest failure by the learner; deficiencies that involve groups of residents point to flaws in the curriculum or its teaching.

Because of the multiple venues and evaluators involved, assessment should be woven carefully into the warp and woof of curricular design, acknowledging practicality as well as content in determining the means of assessment.[8]

Both reliability and validity are critical for assessment of item mastery; however, with the curricular expansion resulting from the addition of core competencies, professional judgment has become an important element in evaluation.

In the development of any assessment system, the following elements should be considered: 1) time availability, since the quality of assessment is related to the time given it; 2) the need for appropriate and specific performance measures; 3) use of multiple evaluators and observations; and 4) the value of application authenticity to determine content validity. The more a simulation approaches clinical reality, the more valid it is. Both video assessments of patient encounters and the use of incognito simulated patients achieve authenticity.

The ACGME has provided a useful template for the development and use of an assessment system, which is summarized in Table 4.1.[9]

TABLE 4.1

Tool	Who evaluates?	How are the evaluators trained?	What performance is evaluated?	How often does this evaluation occur?
Global faculty rating	Faculty	Faculty set behavioral anchors; define meaning of numerical ratings	All 6 competencies All domains	After each rotation
Focused observation	Faculty	Faculty discussion of criteria for patient encounters	Procedural knowledge All 6 competencies All domains	Quarterly
Portfolio	Faculty Mentor Program Director	Faculty establish criteria for portfolio entries	All 6 competencies, especially communication skills and practice-based learning	To be determined
Case logs	Program Director	N/A	Medical knowledge, patient care (quantity), practice-based learning	Semi-annual meeting with Program Director

Tool	Who evaluates?	How are the evaluators trained?	What performance is evaluated?	How often does this evaluation occur?
Cognitive evaluation	Program Director	N/A	Medical knowledge, patient care/skills, sys-based practice	Semi-annual meeting with Program Director
Professional judgment	Faculty	Experientially	All 6 competencies. All domains.	After each rotation

Case logs are useful to document the breadth of clinical experience, and, in some specialties, for credentialing.

Portfolios contribute to self-assessment, goal-setting, and achievement, outlining plans for correcting deficiencies, and summarizing work in progress. By including the resident's own thought and analysis of his or her progress toward professional and personal goals, they also promote introspection and objectivity. Although portfolios are a time-consuming evaluation tool that cannot be scored with numerical precision, they have educational value for the resident, especially if accompanied by mentored feedback.

There are few final or complete answers in medicine, but students are more uncomfortable with uncertainty and ambiguity than with answer A or answer B. Unfortunately, oral and written examinations, which emphasize recall (more important for a physician than recognition) and communication skills, have given way to the ease and "objectivity" of the multiple choice test.

To improve competence testing in medicine, several steps are necessary: competence must be defined by content objectives that are expressed in terms of what the learner must be able to do upon conclusion of the learning experience; and valid and reliable evaluation techniques must be devised that accurately assess the level of achievement.

Some may feel that we are headed in the wrong direction; that what we are really interested in, especially for the practitioner, is performance or incompetence; however, performance is even harder to measure than competence, and having defined the incompetent, we do not yet know what to do with them. Certainly competence does not ensure superior performance, but it is reasonable to assume that one cannot perform adequately without it.

As we continue to search for valid and reliable methods to define and measure competence, we must accept a state of sustained muddle-headedness while the search continues for pieces in a puzzle that will never be complete or perfect. However, since even partial answers to important questions are more useful than complete answers to insignificant ones, the search seems justified.

REFERENCES

1 Mankin JH. Oral examination techniques in the noncognitive domains. In: Lloyd JS, editor. *The Evaluation of Noncognitive Skills and Clinical Performance*. Philadelphia, PA: American Board of Medical Specialties; 1982. pp. 25–31.

2 Lippert FG, Farmer JA. *Psychomotor Skills in Orthopaedic Surgery*. Baltimore, MD: Williams and Wilkins; 1984.

3 Lurie SJ, Mooney CJ, Lyness JM. Measurement of the general competencies of the accreditation council for graduate medical education: a systematic review. *Acad Med*. 2009; **84**(3): 301–8.

4 Brigante RF, Lamb RE. Perception and control test: the dental technical aptitude test of the future? *J Dent Educ*. 1968; **32**(3): 340–54.

5 Louis HJ. Assessment of psychomotor skills. In: Lloyd JS, Langsley DG, editors. *Evaluating the Skills of Medical Specialists*. Philadelphia, PA: American Board of Medical Specialties; 1983, pp. 353–8.

6 Templeton B. Use of interaction analysis in assessing physician trainee interpersonal skills. In: Lloyd JS, editor. *The Evaluation of Noncognitive Skills and Clinical Performance*. Philadelphia, PA: American Board of Medical Specialties; 1982. pp. 155–67.

7 Surdyk PM, Lynch DC, Leach DC. Professionalism: identifying current themes. *Curr Opin Anaesthesiol*. 2003; **16**(6): 597–602.

8 van der Vleuten CPM, Schuwirth LWT. Assessing professional competence: from methods to programs. *Med Educ*. 2005; **39**: 309–17.

9 Joyce B. *Developing an Assessment System: facilitator's guide.* Chicago, IL: Accreditation Council for Graduate Medical Education; 2006. pp. 11–12.

5

Work Hours and the Supervision of Residents*

WORK HOURS

The Accreditation Council for Graduate Medical Education (ACGME) proposed, in their June 1990 revision of the Institutional Requirements, that "Residents should, on average, have at least one 24-hour day out of seven free of patient care responsibilities and should be on call in the hospital no more often than every third night when averaged over a four-week period." They continued by specifying that duty hours must be consistent with the institutional and special requirements that applied to each discipline. An exception to the above standard could be granted "if sufficient reasons exist for a specialty to conduct education with a different method of setting appropriate duty hours" – with the interpretation of "sufficient" and "appropriate" to be made by the ACGME. While these requirements were vetoed initially by the American Board of Medical Specialties (ABMS, a parent of the ACGME), further discussion and clarification led to the adoption in 2003 of specific restrictions on resident work hours, which state that each trainee is limited to a maximum of 30 consecutive work hours, including the time used for sign-out, didactic teaching, and continuity

---

* Parts of this chapter were published in "On work hours for residents," *Annals of Surgery*, 1991; 216(1): 553–4, Lippincott Williams and Wilkins, and "On the supervision of residents," *AOA News*, 1991; **23**: 12. They appear here with the permission of those Journals.

of patient care (the 30-hour rule), and a maximum of 80 weekly work hours, averaged over four weeks (the 80-hour rule). In addition, one day in seven (averaged over four weeks) had to be free of all duties (the seven-day rule). Many disciplines had already revised their special requirements to limit the length of the resident's work week to 80 hours in a humanitarian effort to prevent fatigue and the presumed consequent deterioration in patient care.

Since there is little evidence that duty hour restraints have a measurable effect in preventing medical errors or patient death rates, the implementation of such potentially far-reaching changes was perhaps premature, especially as they emanated from the unfortunate outcome of Libby Zion – an event resulting more from lack of supervision than resident fatigue.[1] If overwork impairs resident performance, it has yet to be shown that the resultant deterioration in patient care is greater than that resulting from "shift medicine."

Acknowledging that residents often work longer hours than trainees in other fields, so too do practicing physicians, who may, when fatigue impairs performance, be harming patients, yet there has been no outcry for limits in this arena. Perhaps the interest in or need for reform does not extend to one's own physician.

And how should a work hour be defined? Is study classified as work? Does being on call, even that part of the night spent sleeping, qualify as work? One definition is time spent in the hospital, in which case, since neither study nor sleep at home would qualify, work becomes as much a matter of venue as activity.

However work is defined, once the principle of limited hours was established, further downward adjustments could be expected.

Among residents in our institution, the number of in-house work hours was found to vary inversely with the number of hours spent in moonlighting activities, and the total work hours did not differ remarkably among disciplines. However, additional pay is received for the moonlighting hours, which may explain, at least in part, the vigor with which limitation of hospital work hours was pursued by organized resident groups. But work is work wherever it occurs, so if the objective is to prevent resident fatigue, moonlighting hours should be the first to go.

Financial constraints have also been cited. Looking at the implementation of similar requirements for New York State, a report in the *Journal of the American Medical Association* estimated additional requirements in excess of $358 million annually and 5358 new positions.[2] If sufficient funding cannot be found, a reduction in resident numbers, salaries, or services would be necessary to be compliant with ACGME regulations.

Broader philosophical questions were also raised by these changes in the Institutional Requirements: is lack of continuity in care a more important determinant of patient outcome than overwork? What is the appropriate body to determine the educational specifics for a given specialty? Should it be that discipline, i.e. the program directors and residency review committees (RRCs), or should it be a general body, which would be less aware of the educational needs for individual specialties?

SUPERVISION

At least as important as work hours in determining patient outcomes is the quality and quantity of resident supervision. Undoubtedly, many errors could be prevented by increased faculty oversight, especially in acute-care venues and of residents at more junior levels. (It might also be that with faculty present, residents would be less often overworked.) Having fewer residents on duty and/or providing care by coverage across services or night floats makes attending coverage even more critical. In one survey of residents, adverse events were related more to insufficient medical supervision (20%) and patient handoffs (13%), than to excessive duty hours (19%).[3]

In large, inner city hospitals especially, residents are frequently called upon to manage complex, acute problems not previously encountered. Faculty may or may not be more than a telephone call away, but calling a more senior person is often equated – overtly or inferentially – with incompetence; so the resident struggles on without benefit of the advice or presence of a more experienced physician. Of course, the reluctance of a resident to ask for help is fostered by the hesitation of a faculty member to come when called, which sends a message about the importance of patient care that outweighs the value of any educational rhetoric.

ISSUES AND OPTIONS

Many of the work-hour issues have been addressed by the ACGME, with the inclusion of sufficient flexibility in the guidelines to accommodate institutional, programmatic and specialty differences, and rapidly evolving clinical events; but the net effect of changing a single variable among the many that determine safe and effective practice will be all but impossible to measure. Nor can it be assumed that more time off can be equated with more sleep rather than moonlighting, housework, or childcare.

Whether or not the period of graduate education will need to be extended is an issue to be considered by each board. Those boards that require specific numbers of procedures may, if the work week is shortened, need a longer educational period, which would increase the costs of GME, or they must require fewer procedures, which, like fatigue, would presumably reduce the quality of patient care.

As the debate on work-hour restrictions continues, further consideration and study should be given to the 30-hour shift length, to a requirement for overlapping coverage, to the effect of work-hour restrictions on learning and experience, and to the difficulty and expense in monitoring 110 000 residents for compliance.

Coverage issues arising from loss of continuity in patient care from "shift medicine" have been addressed at the University of Washington School of Medicine by a computerized sign-out system for resident transition that provides current information on diagnosis, medications and management, allergies, vital signs, lab values, and treatment plan. System efficacy data are not yet available, but anecdotal resident comments suggest improved "hand-off" procedures and patient safety.[4]

With respect to supervision, attending physicians should be assigned to sites of ongoing clinical activity, and the presence of the attending required, so that these assignments are not treated as additional laboratory or desk time. As the federal requirement for the attending physician to see the patient in order to render a charge spread to other third-party carriers, this problem became less of an issue.

Of special concern is supervision on nights and weekends when attendings are not routinely present in the hospital, which is often the time when residents are most fatigued. The answer to this dilemma lies in full-time faculty coverage of the Emergency Department, and the development by each service of specific guidelines for the level of faculty supervision required on nights and weekends.

Supervision of residents takes place at several levels: *direct* supervision exists when faculty are physically present and participate with the resident in providing patient care; *consultative* supervision occurs when faculty provide advice to the resident prior to or during the care of a patient; and *indirect* or retrospective supervision exists when faculty review the care given to a patient by examination of the medical record with the resident. Ideally, faculty supervision should evolve from direct to indirect oversight as the resident becomes more experienced and competent, though the complexity of the problem also influences the level of faculty involvement.

The roles of residents and faculty should be defined in writing by each program, allowing sufficient flexibility for differing clinical circumstances and resident abilities; however, there are principles that guide these policies, including national standards for resident supervision and the need to increase resident responsibility throughout the educational process. Residents should be given freedom to see patients alone and reach decisions regarding diagnosis and management, although final decision-making is the province of the faculty. In general, retrospective review alone is insufficient for first year residents. In emergencies, residents must be permitted to implement life support services, with the attending physician being notified as soon as possible. In critical decision areas, such as the Emergency Department or operating room, there should be direct supervision.

Since evaluation is an integral part of the learning cycle, each resident should be evaluated in writing upon completion of a rotation, along with the resident's progress and performance in the core competencies, and this information forwarded to the program director for appropriate remedial action.

The development of institutional and service guidelines however, does not address fully the frequent attitudinal problem of those residents not wanting supervision, nor that of faculty unwilling to provide it. Residents seek hands-on experience, and faculty members are spread so thin trying to balance all legs of the academic chair that they double up whenever they can. It may be that residents will learn more by trial and error, but this heuristic approach ignores patient outcomes and raises legal and ethical issues. If a resident happens to be one of those unfortunate persons who seems to learn only from his or her own mistakes, the progress of that individual along the educational road will be slow, painful (especially for the patient) and limited. A resident who does not grow through vicarious, as well as his own, experience is potentially dangerous and requires closer monitoring.

Solving attitudinal problems is always difficult. For faculty, the value of supervision should be factored into promotion decisions, since supervision is a critical part of teaching; and documentation of faculty performance should be provided at least annually by anonymous evaluations from the residents being supervised.

Residents must understand that asking for help or guidance is a sign of strength rather than weakness; confident and secure residents are able to say, "I don't know." And of course when they call, someone must answer. Even when the decisions made by residents are not critical, the opportunity to discuss their judgments with someone who has more experience and a broader perspective usually results in more effective patient management, as well as a better learning experience than occurs when such information is proffered in a lecture format – or not at all.

REFERENCES

1 Okie S. An elusive balance – residents' work hours and the continuity of care. *N Engl J Med.* 2007; **356**(26): 2665–7.
2 Thorpe KE. House staff supervision and working hours: implications of regulatory change in New York State. *JAMA.* 1990; **263**: 3177–81.
3 Fletcher KE, Davis SQ, Underwood W, *et al.* Systematic review: effects of resident work hours on patient safety. *Ann Intern Med.* 2004; **141**(11): 851–7.

4 Fuchs E. Residency programs continue to respond to duty hour limits. *AAMC Reporter*. 2008; **18**(1): 5.

6

Science and Service
The Pillars of Professionalism*

Although it may seem out of place for someone so far from the beginning of his career to be addressing those whose professional lives are just emerging, this pattern seems to be rule rather than exception. Perhaps it signifies a search for perspective – for someone who might, by facing backward, enable others to move forward with direction and purpose – analogous to a man rowing a boat who looks to what is past in order to move ahead.

So in searching for a topic, I reflected on those issues that had proved most challenging during my 40-something years in medicine, and was surprised by how often they seemed to have been manifestations of the same generic problems. One was finding a proper balance between thought and action. Many of us, conditioned perhaps by rigorous parental training, came to believe that the highest good lies in action, in doing something. It was a long time before I understood the importance of diastole: that vigorous effort should be alternated with periods of quiet reflection; and that not all movement is forward, nor all change progress.

* Address to the graduating residents, University of Minnesota, June 21, 2002. Parts of this chapter were published in "Medicine in the Third Millenium. What then must we do?" in the *Journal of Bone and Joint Surgery*, 1987; **69A**: 1253–5. They are reprinted here with the permission of that Journal.

It has been necessary to remind myself that lasting monuments were not assembled overnight. Years of labor were required to build the pyramids of Egypt. Civilizations, in fact, are begun in hard work and stoicism; they die Epicurean – in the undisciplined pursuit of individual pleasure and personal convenience.

Another recurrent obstacle – largely a product of specialization – has been the need to sacrifice the horizontal to the vertical dimension. With knowledge in depth, we have purchased ignorance in breadth; in knowing more of parts, we understand less of wholeness.

Also troubling is the relentless ascendancy of fact and technology over principle and precept. A medical fact exists only in the context of a person, and the skill of a physician relates to his or her ability to give that fact appropriate dimension and location within a human being. Method is important in what we do, but in emphasizing techniques, we write upon the water; by instilling principles, we engrave in stone. A mind that understands principles will find its own methods, realizing that technology is a means, not an end. From a full understanding of why, knowledge of what, how, and when proceeds naturally.

Last, and most critical, has been the erosion of professionalism in medicine. Our professionalism reflects our value system. Without it, commitment to the development and maintenance of knowledge and skills, and their use to serve others before self, falters.

Among the core competencies, professionalism is the most critical and among the most difficult to quantify. It is the competency which, possessed in full measure, gives rise to the others. A professional possesses and maintains a unique body of medical knowledge and uses it to provide effective, safe, compassionate, and ethical patient care, including the communication skills necessary to help patients navigate through a complex health care system.

As Cruess and Cruess have pointed out, the place of physicians in a contemporary, complex society is determined by the degree to which they fulfill the related roles as healer and as professional.[1] Healing is well taught during medical school and residency; the other area of accountability – professionalism – which protects and informs the role of the healer, has received relatively little formal attention.

As physician-healers moved medicine from superstition to science, professionalism, evolving from the Hippocratic Oath, blended with the healing arts as a modulating influence.[1]

As its unique body of knowledge and skills expanded, medicine became more autonomous and preoccupied with its own needs and benefits, rather than those of society in general – with avarice rather than altruism, which is responsible for much of the current criticism of the profession.

A development that followed World War II, the corporatization of medicine, has made the state and marketplace major players in the provision of health care. As a result, the corporate sector, with its profit-based *modus operandi*, became by the 1990s the dominant player in the delivery of health care – diminishing the role of physicians and professional organizations.

Medicine must respond to these challenges; how it does so will determine its future place in society. Doing nothing is not a choice.

Although the long definition of the word "profession" contains many elements, professionalism is founded on the pillars of science and service, upon possession of a specialized body of knowledge and skills, and the obligation to use that expertise to serve others before self. The relationship between service to public and service to self has always been a delicate balance. A profession is clearly a career, a vocation; as such, one may expect to earn a living from its pursuit. But more central to the idea of a profession is the obligation of its members to value altruism above reward. Perhaps the best way to visualize the relationship between the two is to consider service the obligation of professionals and reward their privilege.

At the heart of this obligation is ethics, and at the heart of ethics is the welfare of the patient. Medical ethics unfolded from the principles of individual behavior laid down in the Hippocratic Oath, into a broader context that includes responsibility of the profession to self-regulate, access to care, cost-effectiveness, and prevention. The ethical conflict produced by the obligation of a physician to both the patient (for whom quality care is paramount) and the employer (for whom cost containment and profit are the dominant forces) led to the insertion of third parties between physicians and their patients.

How this conflict between cost and care is resolved will determine whether medicine retains its high position among the professions. Our personal values will determine the ethical plane on which medicine is practiced.

In the past, physicians determined how care was delivered; now lawyers, bureaucrats, other health professionals, insurers, and patients have their own concept of medicine. As these interpretations multiply and diverge, the search for a unifying ethos becomes more critical and more difficult.

Physicians must also deal with conflict in their personal value systems. Consider, for example, the tension between the physician's roles as healer and as scientist. As healer one is expected to act in the best interest of the individual patient; as scientist, the physician must respect the precepts of valid clinical trials, which may prove to be suboptimal treatment of some patients to ensure optimal therapy for all patients.

Changing societal perceptions have also created ethical controversies. The current notion that blame must be fixed for anything less than a perfect result has led to an unfair tort system and astronomical malpractice rates. While the distinction between unfortunate and unreasonable outcomes is often blurred, these judgments must be made; and clearly others, including patients themselves, must assume outcome responsibility. A person dies not just of a disease but also of his or her entire life.

ISSUES AND OPTIONS

Hearing less about care and suffering and more about costs and bottom lines, residents today see medicine more as a business than a calling; in fact, the major threat to the ethos of professionalism in medicine is what Hafferty has identified as "rampant commercialism." Deplored and decried 20 years ago, commercialism today is passed off as "the way things are." The author cited self- and peer review as more critical in solving these professional issues than the policies of institutions and organizations.[2]

Contributing to the pervasiveness of commercialism are the conflicts of interest between medicine and industry. Collaborations between academia and industry have often been productive and beneficial; but gift-giving and underwriting professional meetings for those positioned to influence the sales of their products have – given the natural inclination toward reciprocity – raised ethical issues. Does industry's largesse influence clinical judgment, reporting of research findings, or the use of drugs and medical devices produced by a sponsoring company? Probably. Clearly, organized medicine and institutions must study and clarify policies and procedures that govern these relationships to maintain public trust in the integrity of medical research and education.

In June 2008, the AAMC issued recommendations on conflict of interest prohibiting all gifts of food, calling for central management of product samples, restricting industry representatives' access to physicians, and distributing CME funds from a central medical center office. Deans and faculty members have taken the lead in developing new institutional policies, insisting that science and need, rather than marketing, drive decision-making, with the goal being a change in the ethos of an institution from a sense of personal entitlement toward an obligation to science, society, and patients.[3]

Most solutions create their own set of problems, and technological answers to medical problems have been no exception. The eruption of procedural methodologies has created a bewildering array of choices that did not exist previously. Consider the ethical dilemmas posed by our increased capacity to extend life and our commitment to relieve suffering; or by our ability to enhance the quality of life and the obligation to conserve resources – especially when we see technology used with more benefit to physician reimbursement than health care.

What then should be done to preserve the ethical dimension that accounts for medicine's distinction as a profession – to resolve the deepening conflicts between personal and public interests; between our obligation to provide optimal care and economic constraints; between the best treatment and the patient's right to decide; or between the physician as healer and the physician as scientist? As ballast for these increasingly turbulent waters, we must rededicate ourselves to the fundamental values of medicine.

First, the patient's welfare must be given highest priority. To the extent that we become brokers for third parties rather than advocates for patients, we sacrifice the public trust so critical to the high position that medicine has held in the past; but we can no longer ignore economic considerations in health care decisions. Medical resources, like the grass in a pasture, are limited. It may seem harmless enough to add a few private cows to the medical pasture, but if everyone acts in the same manner, the medical commons will soon be exhausted. Irresponsible individual action can thus decimate the entire medical community. By applying the principle of universality – that is, by stopping to consider the consequences of personal action becoming a universal mode of behavior – the inherent propriety of an act may be better understood.

We must also realize that it is perfectly acceptable for a patient to refuse a specific recommendation for therapy, even if this decision does not seem to be in his or her best interest, provided the patient has sufficient knowledge and awareness to make an informed decision. There is no reason for a terminally ill patient to be maintained indefinitely as a heart-lung preparation, which, like pasting summer leaves on winter trees, is unseemly as well as impractical.

Finally, we must await reliable epidemiologic data before treatments are adopted for widespread use. It may be argued that failure to employ intuitively or anecdotally effective therapy denies or delays optimal care, but the medical roadside is littered with abandoned therapies whose initial use was suggested by judgment or logic – remember gastric freezing for peptic ulcers, the "button" operation for ascites, and frontal lobotomies. After wide dissemination, such procedures are not easily withdrawn – even by an author with the integrity to debunk his own inventions. By testing the efficacy of new treatment, science can be lifted from the fog of empiricism. To accomplish these ends, to make physicians aware of the obligations that accompany professional status, the education of medical students and residents must inculcate the belief that professional behavior is essential for the healer to function properly in contemporary society.

Recognizing medical education as an apprenticeship that includes the dimensions of understanding, skill acquisition, and the use of knowledge and skills to serve patients and society, Cruess and Cruess have argued persuasively for a curriculum in professionalism to establish the bedrock of medical education, with standard means of assessment to determine the learner's commitment to and progress toward these goals.[4]

Parker, *et al.* have described a program that integrates medical ethics, law, and professionalism into a curriculum for personal and professional development. Reporting on over 500 students who completed this program between 2000 and 2006, they demonstrated that even a large medical school could meet the challenges of teaching and assessing the noncognitive domain. Student mastery of the formal curriculum was determined through written tests and objective structured clinical examinations, with the addition of an assessment process for attitudes and behaviors.[5]

In receiving baccalaureate degrees, students join the company of educated men and women. As graduate trainees, they enter the community of professionals, which, unlike other communities, has no solitary locus or language and worships at no single shrine. It is, rather, an imagined community, one that is steadily defined and redefined by discourse and action and maintained by our faith in it. Accompanying sound clinical knowledge and judgment must be the values that sustain society. Loss of autonomy will occur if medicine neglects its obligations to society as a whole. There will be new and demanding challenges to conducting oneself with integrity. In order to manage complex tasks, we will be tempted to dissemble or to take intellectual and personal shortcuts; but medicine is a very special kind of human endeavor, one that cannot be pursued effectively without humility, integrity, compassion, and the effacement of self-interest. We must not succumb to pressures to become commercial entrepreneurs, gate-closers, or agents of any fiscal policy that runs counter to the public trust and our concern for the primacy of the patient's well-being.

While physician ownership of the medical world may be questioned, especially if we accept the Biblical statement that "the earth is the Lord's and the fullness thereof," we are, even in this context, the stewards of medicine. There is admittedly some unfairness in this arrangement, since we have been given something we did not ask for or create; but this has been true for every generation of physicians who preceded us, and it will be the lot of those that follow.

We can only hope that those who do not feel a sense of ownership and responsibility will be outdone by those who do. If the former group predominates, we should begin searching for another Gibbon – for someone to record the decline and fall of this era of civilization, for, as previous civilizations have shown us, whenever consumption exceeds production, that civilization eventually disappears. Waste is thus an ancestor of poverty.

Never again will we occupy this space and time; it has been given us in trust. Certainly a wind is rising and strong currents are flowing around the pillars of science and service. Whether they can withstand these forces of change will depend in large measure upon our adherence to high standards of practice. If we drop below that level or violate ethical and moral trusts, if we are avaricious or allow technology to replace rather than complement personal involvement, we will have surrendered medicine to the tides of change. Noble purposes are fragile and easily overcome by materialistic concerns; in the end, however, it is the placement of giving in front of taking that will make the difference. If we respect this order, the quality of medical care will endure, and medicine will retain its place of honor at the professional table.

REFERENCES

1 Cruess RL, Cruess SR. Teaching medicine as a profession in the service of healing. *Acad Med.* 1997; **72**(11): 941–2.

2 Hafferty F. The elephant in medical professionalism's kitchen. *Acad Med.* 2006; **81**(10): 906–14.

3 Rothman DJ, Chimonas S. New developments in managing physician-industry relationships. *JAMA.* 2008; **300**(9): 1067–9.

4 Cruess RL, Cruess SR, Steinert Y. *Teaching Medical Professionalism.* New York, NY: Cambridge University Press; 2009.

5 Parker M, Luke H, Zhang J, *et al.* The "pyramid of professionalism": seven years of experience with an integrated program of teaching, developing, and assessing professionalism among medical students. *Acad Med.* 2008; **83**(8): 733–41.

7

No Tempests, No Teapots
Fostering Research in Medical Education[*]

I should perhaps explain this title. When asked for a topic before deciding on a subject – let alone what to call it – there was much more room to say what it was *not* than what it *was* about, so it seemed safer to title it "No Tempests, No Teapots," since I did not plan to cover either of those subjects.

Reflecting on the importance of the residency years to our professional lives, my thoughts went back to the origin of graduate medical education at the Johns Hopkins Hospital in the late 1800s, when the term *resident* was coined from the expectation that junior physicians would reside in the hospital on essentially a full-time basis. The enormous expansion of this educational domain since, both in breadth and depth, is a tribute to the creative insights of Osler, Halsted, and Welch, who perceived its great value to both learner and teacher.

Explosive growth, however, is never trouble-free, and graduate medical education has been no exception. Supervision, work hours,

---

[*] Address to the Thirty-Second Annual Orthopaedic Residents' Conference of the American Orthopaedic Association, Chapel Hill, North Carolina, March 12, 1999. Parts of this address were published in "Creativity in Medicine" in *Symbols and Symptoms*. Indianapolis, IN: Guild Press; 1995, and *The Journal of Bone and Joint Surgery*. 1999; **81**(A): 1205–8. It appears here with the permission of that Journal.

funding, the balance between service and education, and territorial disputes are issues that have defied complete or final answers. Another issue, especially germane to graduate training, is the role of research in the education of residents. Many disciplines with excellent clinical and educational programs have not had a commensurate impact in research. Partial justification for this shortcoming may lie in the heavy clinical responsibilities of the discipline. However – and this is my thesis – some capacity for creation exists in everyone, and the enhancement of this creative potential is not only possible but also a necessary and proper function of all who participate in the education of physicians.

Creativity has been variously interpreted. Broadly defined, it is bringing something new into existence by recognizing a relationship between previously unassociated elements. Implicit in this definition is a product, and the notion that human creation results not *ex nihilo* but from the use of existing material in unusual ways.

Creative people tend to prepare themselves, consciously or unconsciously, for discovery through three steps: 1) personal interest in a topic; 2) study and thought (often illuminated by a sudden idea); and 3) by the formulation and testing of a hypothesis.

Curiosity is a prime requisite for a career of exploration. It has been condemned as a condition that kills, and theologians have testified that it cost us paradise; nevertheless, curiosity is the mainspring of seekers, of people who want to know. Creative individuals are also more likely to be observant, sensitive, persistent, and to possess the capacity for intense concentration, a high tolerance for ambiguity, and the faculty for divergent thought. Divergent thought, which enables one to perceive similarities among previously dissimilar elements, is more critical to the creative process than convergent thought, which depends on recall and application of learned material. Aptitude for convergent thought and high intelligence are frequently associated. However, above an intelligence quotient of 120, creativity has not been shown to be related to intelligence.[1]

Further shape may be given to the concept of creativity by understanding what it is not. For example, the simple enumeration of facts increases our knowledge but produces no remarkable insight or novel design. By counting, one may determine the number of seeds in an apple, thereby obtaining factual information, but, by determining the number of apples in a seed, one obtains knowledge of greater moment.

Likewise, the simple act of discovery is not creation. Finding an apple that has fallen from a tree is not creative, but by connecting the forces that caused the apple to fall with those required to keep the moon in its orbit, Newton made an inductive leap that is the essence of creativity.

Finally, it is important to distinguish creation from interpretation. Although the renowned actor may receive more acclaim than the author of the play, it is the latter who created the piece in which the actor performs, however skillfully.

Creativity has both vertical and horizontal dimensions. The vertical plane encompasses the levels of creativity, ranging from simple, expressive originality (a clever phrase or a new dance movement) to complex forms of abstraction. Between the expressive and abstract levels is innovation, wherein the application of known principles, devices, or information provides a better way of doing something, of controlling the world around us.

The horizontal dimension embraces the types of creativity. Although the urge to create is largely independent of professional training, creation in artistic fields differs from that in science by having a smaller canon of technology and fact between the creative spark and its expression. Thus, artistic creation is less influenced by conscious thought than is scientific discovery, although the flash of illumination that springs from the well of subconscious cerebration occurs in both. The "Eureka!" of Archimedes as he stepped into the bathtub resulted from a spontaneous apposition of thought and inspiration similar to that which produced a Shakespearean sonnet. Such inductive leaps, however, being intuitive, are sometimes wrong. In science, the generalizations that result must be followed by hypothesis and experiment – the scientific method – which entail conscious connections, logic, and analytic thought.

It is then a blend of inspiration and analysis that has produced the peaks of creative achievement in medicine. We may be justly proud of past accomplishments, but a steady decline of physician-investigators clouds the future of medical discovery. That the causes for this decline are not based on genetic incompetence was suggested by Gough, whose studies showed that medical students had greater creative potential than did architects, engineers, mathematicians, and research scientists.[2] External influences probably start much earlier than we realize – perhaps the first time that we offer a child an ice-cream cone as a reward for building a sand castle, and, by this careless introduction to the marketplace, encourage him or her to work for external rewards rather than for the inner pleasure of doing.

Further discouragement often occurs in elementary school, where to be different is to be disorderly or disruptive. The need for structure and discipline encourages convergent rather than divergent behavior. Exceptional sensitivity and skill are required of a teacher to preserve classroom order and simultaneously allow creative minds to expand. The student who, when asked to draw a house, depicts its inside rather the expected outside should be praised, not criticized, for this deviation from the ordinary.

Another characteristic of those bent toward medicine, whether innate or acquired, is a hypertrophied work ethic. While the essentiality and value of hard work are undeniable, continued focus on the next course or the next patient reduces the time for free association and creative thought. This preoccupation with task completion – with becoming rather than being – narrows perspective; other dimensions disappear. An initially diverse group of medical students, homogenized by traditional forms of language, practice, and dress, come to sound, act, and look alike.

Embryological research has shown that organisms act *on* their environment before reacting *to* it, so perhaps the inclination to work is congenital[3]. But creativity, like many natural phenomena, is a cyclic process in which effort and relaxation, work and play, are balanced. Unfortunately, our culture equates relaxation with idleness, perceiving it more as a reward for work than its necessary diastole. However, unrelieved activity has an undesirable side effect: it reduces the time for wonder, for understanding the world around us, and for seeing the unusual in the ordinary.

Even nonprofessional pastimes tend toward competitive and self-improvement modes. We are supposed to be producing something, making things add up, getting ahead. Doing nothing is not easy; it takes courage and intelligence of a high order, and it takes practice. Of course, the more one does it, the easier it gets, and, after a while, even the guilt subsides.

Creativity is further constrained by the educational experience. The traditional authoritarianism of medicine, an enormous amount of factual material, and the pervasive multiple-choice test encourage a black-or-white, yes-or-no type of thought that allows little room for ambiguity. No one relishes intellectual purgatory, but we must realize that some questions have many answers and others none, and understand that uncertainty and anxiety are inevitable, and therefore acceptable, emotions. Perhaps, as Cohen suggested, we should have uncertainty rounds that deal only with patients whose problems have no single or best answer.[4]

After completing graduate education, most physicians enter practice, where stereotypical behavior is fostered by societal expectations and peer pressure. Others become faculty members, and their creative lives become emasculated by bureaucratic detail, Sisyphean labors, and the quest for elusive grant support. To be successful in today's world, the medical scientist must be not only a thinker but also a worker and perhaps a miser. Of course, if confusion is a condition of creativity, the university environment is more asset than impediment.

ISSUES AND OPTIONS

To protect the future of medicine, all medical schools and GME disciplines should have curricular requirements for education in research methodology, interpretation, and ethics, and the opportunity to participate in research projects. They must understand that research is important not just for the sake of doing, but because it results in better patient care.

The first step is to identify those who are unusually imaginative, since the innovative applicant is not set apart by present methods of selection. Psychometric indices of creativity could be incorporated into the Medical College Aptitude Test or the Scholastic Aptitude Test.

The critical incident technique might also be used to identify students possessing the traits most often associated with creative behaviors.

We must also insist on greater undergraduate diversity so students can maintain their horizontal dimension as long as possible. Verticality will come soon enough. Although facts are the raw material of ideas, research is more than collecting data. Perspective shapes the content of observation, and, to the extent that perspective is rooted in worldview, science is informed by nonscience.

Special emphasis should be given to college courses that stress concepts and principles, logic and analysis, and metaphoric activity. Both analytic and metaphoric processes are needed by the creative scientist. Analysis divides, categorizes, and emphasizes differences; metaphor relates, unites, and stresses similarities. Philosophy is vital because it encourages analysis and discipline and, above all, a search for truth. And, lest we forget, a course in expository writing so that the rest of us will not have to hack our way through the seemingly obligatory obfuscation of medical writing.

After the native inventiveness and intellectual breadth of a student are ensured, the spark should be fanned by exposure to role models who reflect their enjoyment of research, and by providing time free from clinical responsibilities. But a neophyte investigator should not simply be taken off the wards and told to "do some research." Direction is critical in framing the questions for study and in planning the experiments to test hypotheses generated by these questions. Considerable experience and knowledge of the field are necessary to set in place the other pieces of the puzzle that determine the size and shape of those being sought.

A research project is likely to bear fruit in proportion to the investigator's powers of observation, objectivity, and patience. Accurate observation depends on a receptive mind. It is easy to overlook the unfamiliar, whereas one readily perceives the familiar. We are often prone to see what lies behind our eyes rather than what appears before them.

Objectivity entails the honest acceptance of data that arise in the course of investigation, even if it results in the slaying of a beautiful hypothesis by an ugly fact.

Patience is essential to enable the investigator to surmount the tangle of hindrances that lie invariably in his or her path. Occasionally, overcoming these obstacles gives rise to results as important as those originally sought. Of course, there is always the possibility that what has been imagined cannot be proven by available means, in which case persistence becomes foolish – what Emerson called "the hobgoblin of little minds."

Nascent researchers must understand too that if, as often happens, the research period produces no "Eureka!" experiences, the enhanced appreciation of scientific methods, and the ability to examine with a more critical eye are justifiable outcomes. House officers should have opportunities to present their preliminary work for analysis and comment in seminars and research meetings, with the expectation that the final paper will reach a national forum and/or publication.

One avenue for medical students who aspire to careers as research scientists is the MD/PhD program offered by about 40 medical schools. These programs are supported by the National Institute of General Medical Sciences and provide a stipend, tuition, allowance, and other educational expenses. After two years of medical school, students typically spend at least the next three years in their PhD programs, then re-enter medical school for the last two years of study for the MD degree, followed by three to five years in their clinical specialty; but spending five to seven clinical years before embarking in earnest on their research careers places them at a competitive disadvantage for NIH funding. Data cited by Whitcomb indicates that fewer than half of the graduates of these programs become independently funded investigators.[5] Critical to the success of these programs is more complete integration of the requirements for the PhD into the period when graduates are involved in advanced clinical training.

Another option for those who wish to include research in their careers is to extend their education in translational research, perhaps to the level of a master's degree, which would, either as an integrated or an additional period of education, have minimal impact on the total length of training and would partner naturally with clinical practice and teaching.

Many physicians, hearing the term "translational research," think simply of the transfer of laboratory research to the bedside, but it also includes the transmission and integration of results from clinical studies into everyday practice patterns. Translational research thus offers research opportunities ranging from molecular science and biotechnology to epidemiology and systems analysis, for each of which there are different goals, strategies, and research settings.

Recognizing translational research as a viable and highly practical means of applying progress in the biological sphere to the improvement of health care, the NIH has established centers for translational research within its institutes and initiated the Clinical and Translational Science Award program (CTSA), encouraging other federal and state agencies and academic institutions to do the same. As of 2008, 38 academic health centers had earned a CTSA from the NIH. The establishment of approximately 60 CTSAs was anticipated by 2012, with an annual budget of $500 million, although prospects for this level of funding have been jeopardized by the current economic downturn.[6] CTSAs are expected to develop active networking among major academic research centers and strong engagement with their local communities.

Although a positive experience is more likely if the interest and enthusiasm of the investigator are captured in the project, it does not matter greatly whether the research is in basic or applied science if the problems are addressed through rigorous application of the scientific method. The axiom that basic research is needed to advance the understanding of clinical medicine brooks no credible opposition. Although the border between clinical research and fundamental science is sometimes blurred, groundbreaking innovation may come from either. The health of the fruit is closely tied to that of the tree that bears it. The ways of looking at problems are, or should be, very much the same whether one is engaged in research or in practice. The scientific method is for both a conduit to the summit of professionalism, the creation of new knowledge. We cannot create from nothingness, which must be left to a higher being, but may we not hope, as in the majestic passage from *The Divine Comedy*, for the power to leave "one spark of God's glory to the race to come?"[7]

REFERENCES

1 Vernon PE. *Creativity*. Baltimore, MD: Penguin; 1970.

2 Gough HG. What happens to creative medical students? *J Med Educ*. 1976; **51**(6): 461–7.

3 Piontelli A. Twins: from fetus to child. London: Routledge; 2002.

4 Cohen ML. Uncertainty rounds. *JAMA*. 1983; **250**(13): 1689.

5 Whitcomb ME. The need to restructure MD-PhD training. *Acad Med*. 2007; **82**(7): 623–4.

6 Woolf SH. The meaning of translational research and why it matters. JAMA. 2008; **299**(2): 211–13.

7 Dante. *The Divine Comedy*. Garden City, NY: Doubleday; 1947.

8

Psychomotor Education
Point and Counterpoint*

There is little room for argument with the notion that much of what is highest and best in medicine has resulted from advances in technology. One need only consider the diagnostic power of magnetic resonance imaging and the therapeutic impact of surgical miniaturization to realize the claim of technology on medical care. Nor is this debt limited to the direct management of disease. Through technological adaptation, the computer has created the science of information management, which has become an indispensable adjunct to health care. Students grow up with high-definition television and interactive programming; in fact, with journals and textbooks accessible from the television screen, the classroom may shift to the home, spawning a new type of faculty career: the professorial media star.

Given this level of wiring, it should not be surprising that technology and its associated financial rewards have tilted surgical education toward "hows" rather than "whys," toward technique rather than understanding. In addition, more time in the operating room has reduced preoperative and postoperative patient contact, which also is critical to operative outcomes. A patient's understanding, expectations, and needs must be explored and clarified before operative

* This chapter was published in a slightly different text in *The Journal of Bone and Joint Surgery*. 1993; **75**(9): 1263–4 and was reprinted in *The Iowa Orthopaedic Journal*. 1994; **14**: 106–7. It is reprinted here with the permission of that Journal.

intervention; and extended monitoring after surgery may be necessary to determine long-term outcomes, which cannot be predicted at the time of suture removal.

The formal teaching of motor skills was initiated in Orthopaedics by Lippert and others whose whip-and-chair efforts not only tamed the curricular tiger but also established the utility of motor-skills laboratories for the education of orthopaedic surgeons.[1] However, as they noted, successful surgery entails more than manual dexterity. Precise and complete separation of motor skills from thought and subjective response is neither possible nor desirable; hands are the servants of heart and head. In addition to coordinated and efficient movement, a surgeon should possess equanimity, confidence, perseverance, flexibility, and the capacity for honest self-appraisal – all tempered by a basic reluctance to operate. Essential cognitive attributes include knowledge of disease and patient and of operative and non-operative alternatives, the capacity for logical thought, and the ability to anticipate.

Knowledge of the effectiveness of a procedure is of particular importance. If there is no indication for an operation, there is no indication for doing it well. The collision between proliferating health care technology and cost-containment has stimulated intense public and legislative scrutiny of procedural interventions; as a result, funding limitations will be increasingly restricted to procedures with documented effectiveness, which will reduce the number of operative interventions for the treatment of effects rather than causes. The employment of arthroscopy, for example, to shave the retropatellar surface, can be challenged by the failure to document long-term cost-effectiveness. In seeking such documentation, we may find that shaving is less appropriate for the patella than for the face, where, as befits cosmetic operations, its effects may be more readily perceived.

ISSUES AND OPTIONS
The rapid development of procedural tools has created a bewildering panoply of choices that did not exist previously, and the relationship between the use of technology and reimbursement levels has

increased the costs of medical care, raised ethical issues, and too often made technology an end rather than a means. In the educational arena, more powerful educational tools have shifted the emphasis toward process rather than purpose and content of education.

Departmental names, boundaries, and teaching responsibilities have become blurred by the inclusion of high-tech molecular and cell biology orientations, which has increased the potential for curricular gaps and redundancies.

Sophisticated technology has given medical education computer-assisted instruction, virtual simulations, and computerized mannequins. Shorter hospital stays and the reduced opportunities for students to encounter infrequent but important clinical events make these alternatives valuable educational tools, particularly for teaching surgery, since mistakes are not associated with increased morbidities. They also provide a means of meeting the requirements of accrediting bodies for numbers of procedures or instruction in the core competencies. Using images or models alone to study the structure of body parts is, however, somewhat like exploring a city with a guidebook rather than walking the streets oneself. It also uncovers one of the age-old dilemmas of medical care: striking a proper balance between too little and too much personal involvement with patients. Learning on simulators pushes the learner toward detachment; but dissection in the anatomy laboratory – realizing that a total stranger has given his or her last full measure to advance the learning of others – stirs empathy. Thus, replacing gross anatomy dissections with computerized simulations may have greater professional cost than benefit. There will always be a need for the inspiration and individual attention provided by personal interaction between teacher and learner.

The impact of technology has also been felt in research. The emergence of molecular mechanisms as the explanation of many diseases has, by creating a gap between research and bedside, contributed to the decline of clinical teaching; and the movement toward reductionism has directed investigation away from issues of lifestyle, environment, and social needs.

Most treatments benefit symptoms, but only through double-blinded, randomized studies will we know which treatments alter the course of a disease. Achilles tenotomy may relieve claudication but could hardly be considered appropriate treatment for ischemic disease. Neither unaudited experience nor logical thought can replace controlled clinical trials, so until documentation of a procedure's effectiveness can be demonstrated, it should be considered a false idol and worship withheld. Unfortunately, the stimulus response model still heavily influences American education; if a new instrument or procedure is offered, it is adopted. By using valid outcome studies, however, physicians can avoid seduction by anecdotal reports from so-called authorities whose numerators are still in search of denominators.

In spite of the growing tendency to equate surgery solely with procedural events, surgery is more than the sum of its operations; and neither the existence of an instrument nor the ability to perform an operation adeptly is an indication for surgical intervention.

In addition to honing manual skills, psychomotor education should cultivate an understanding that new is not better until it is proved to be so. The medical roadside is littered with technologies that not only failed to improve patients but harmed them; indeed, the initial enthusiasms for bloodletting, frontal lobotomy, and gastric freezing should give us pause to consider which of our current procedures will lie with these relics as the follies of our time.

While there is no single correct answer to the question of how much time should be purchased from other educational domains to teach manual skills, preoccupation with technique should not replace time spent listening to, looking at, or examining the patient. By permitting the technical aspects of education to erode other essential clinical skills, the humanistic base of medical practice will be diminished. It should also be remembered that cognitive aspects of surgical procedures can be taught in skills laboratories as well as motor and technical skills.

The foregoing concerns over the potential for abuse of technology are meant neither to devalue the importance of technologic advances, nor to take a mean view of technical training in general. There is natural pleasure and benefit in doing, in applying knowledge and thought to produce tangible products that satisfy practical needs. The union of theory and practice is an integral part of a well-rounded education.

Technological prowess can help to begin life, delay death, cure cancer, and repair or replace critical parts, but unless it is integrated harmoniously with the heart and head of a physician, modern medicine will fail to maintain a humanitarian counterpoint to the anvil chorus of technology.

REFERENCE

1 Lippert FG, Farmer JA. *Psychomotor Skills in Orthopaedic Surgery*. Baltimore, MD: Williams and Wilkins; 1984.

9

Teaching by Residents

Passing It On*

Qui docent discet – *Those who teach, learn*

Reports on the role of residents as teachers have appeared in the medical literature for more than 30 years citing improvement in the knowledge and interactive skills of residents in addition to benefits to students.[1,2,3] It has been estimated that at any given time, approximately 100 000 residents are working alongside half the nation's medical students, who will obtain 20–70% of their clinical teaching from these residents.[4,5,6,7] Being frontline clinical contacts for students, residents must be committed and competent teachers.

Teaching by residents traditionally complements that of attending physicians: clinical principles taught by faculty in lecture formats are applied in the context of patient care, where resident–student interaction is common. Residents are effective teachers in these settings because they focus on practical aspects of care and understand the needs of students. They often are better suited, for example, to teaching basic technical skills than staff members who have become less conscious of the individual steps needed by the novice to master a

* Published in a slightly different format in *Journal of Bone and Joint Surgery (Am)*. 2001; **83**: 1441–3. Parts of this chapter were published in *Clinical Orthopaedics and Related Research*. 2007; **454**: 247–50. It appears here with the permission of Lippincott Williams and Wilkins.

given procedure. Being closer in age, the near peer status of residents makes them more approachable for "stupid questions" than members of the faculty.

Not surprisingly, medical students who are exposed to highly rated instructors (faculty and residents) during a clinical rotation are more likely to pursue that discipline. In one study, 9 of 29 students who had worked with a "best" clinical instructor chose that field for residency, whereas 0 of 23 equally well-qualified students who worked with a "worst" instructor did so.[8]

ISSUES AND OPTIONS

Because teaching by residents is crucial to the education of the student and teacher, the issue is not whether residents should teach, but how they can do it more effectively. There are at least six impediments to more proficient teaching by residents,[3] each of which is remediable.

1 Inadequate role modeling

Lack of faculty commitment to the teaching enterprise is perhaps the major obstacle to improving the enthusiasm, effort, and teaching skills of residents. Too often, teaching, especially of medical students, is an optional rather than a required faculty responsibility. Teaching students should be a requirement by the school, for promotion, with participation by all departmental members. A strong argument can be made that teaching students is the most important obligation for medical school faculty; if they are not enthusiastic, competent, and accessible teachers of medical students, it is unrealistic to require or expect those qualities in residents. Residents must see clear evidence of faculty commitment to education, which, in one form or another, should be manifest in all activities of the department.

Quantifiable means of measuring teaching effectiveness, such as the Relative Value Metrics System developed by the Association of American Medical Colleges, are available to promotions committees.[9]

2 Time and monetary constraints

As the influence of the marketplace on health care has increased, teaching hospitals, whose mission includes a heavy educational component, have become disadvantaged.[10] With medical school budgets more dependent on clinical revenue, and reimbursement decreasing for each unit of service, clinical faculty have been compelled to spend more time in patient care, often at the expense of teaching time.

The compression of teaching time has created a need for greater efficiency. Complete separation of work and teaching rounds, for example, may be impractical, but by simply thinking aloud as decisions are made during work rounds, residents can make education a valuable by-product. Additional teaching time may be found during night and weekend call activities when residents are working one-on-one with students. Coffee breaks and down time between patients and/or operating room cases provide other "teachable moments" which, being out of the earshot of patients, are also useful occasions for feedback to students. Every encounter involving a resident and a student should be viewed as an opportunity to teach and, more importantly, to demonstrate nonverbal professional attitudes and behaviors.

We can and should make more efficient use of teaching opportunities, but given the strong link between time and money, we also must confront the more formidable task of providing salary support for faculty time dedicated to teaching. The scientific community has risen to the challenge of protecting the biomedical research agenda. In similar fashion, we should make clear to institutional and national funding sources the critical importance of strong support for medical education to assure the future of medical practice.

As a related thought, since teaching time is often at the expense of research time, why not direct some of our research into innovative educational efforts?

3 Lack of instruction in the principles of adult education and techniques of teaching

Because it defines us as professionals and as individuals, teaching is too important to be delegated to residents without guidance. Morrison, *et al.* showed a considerable difference in teaching effectiveness between internal medicine residents who had a 13-hour interventional program to improve their teaching skills and a control group. Residents were required to attend. Evaluation/feedback, teacher behavior, and discussion leader skills were the topics receiving greatest curricular emphasis. The intervention residents also manifested greater enthusiasm for teaching, more learner-centered approaches, and a fuller understanding of teaching principles and skills.[11] Another study evaluated the effect of a six-hour course on resident teaching and leadership skills.[12] The authors analyzed three years of resident teaching evaluations before and after the introduction of a teaching skills course using a standardized teaching assessment form. Mean ratings showed continuous and statistically significant improvement each year after the introduction of the course.

In a survey of internal medicine programs, 20% had programs to improve resident teaching skills.[2] The mean instructional time was nine hours, with a range of 1–24 hours. Half of the programs required resident attendance. Although the curriculum was not standardized, the use of evaluation/feedback as a teaching tool was the topic most commonly covered in the teaching sessions.

A teacher-training program for residents must prepare them to teach the essential skills of history taking, physical examination, and basic technical procedures. In the study by Bing-You and Harvey, the three major factors that correlated with teaching effectiveness were: active involvement of the students, accessibility, and demonstration of clinical skills and procedures.[1] Residents must also be prepared to help students in their assessment of the medical literature so that students may ground their practice decisions in evidence-based data. They must also understand the importance of an empathetic attitude, nonthreatening feedback, and time management. Successful residents provide constructive feedback and create an educational environment that encourages learning by coupling knowledge with enthusiasm and personal commitment.

Valid instruments are available to assess the effectiveness of resident teaching, including objective structured teaching examinations and rating scales, which include narrative feedback from the medical students. Written feedback is more valuable than oral for improving resident performance and increasing resident interest in teaching.[13]

For motivated adults, the principal determinants of learning are active involvement of the learner and problem-centered teaching; nonjudgmental feedback and the opportunity for repetition are critical adjuncts.[14] Surgical residents, whose time for patient interaction with students is limited by the demands of the operating room, are understandably prone to an authoritative approach emphasizing recall and delivery of facts, sometimes forgetting that too much information can obscure the learning process. Although an assertive style sometimes is useful, teaching only by force-feeding information – by faculty or residents – like the proverbial Strasbourg goose, produces a pâté that contains too much of the formulaic and too little of the ethos of medicine. We persist in teaching facts, even though learning based on understanding and reflection is more likely to be stored in long-term memory because it is easier to impart information than to teach students how to think.

Even experienced instructors sometimes forget that teaching does not ensure learning. It is a mistake to consider teachers the active and students the passive participants in education. Students must realize that the primary responsibility for their education rests with them. Both parties must be active for learning to occur, so interactive teaching and independent learning should increase as the trainee moves through the educational continuum.

Teaching techniques vary with content, venue, and group size. Small-group teaching differs from the lecture format by delivering content in small bites based on data generated from a patient, and by opportunities to display collaborative, motor, and attitudinal behaviors more frequently.

Clinic and bedside teaching enable students to perceive the critical role of a humanistic dimension in increasingly technologic methods of care. By reflecting caring and concern, residents serve as positive role models for students, and by coming quickly to the essence of a problem, the resident can show how efficient time management can coexist with respect and empathy. In their preoccupation with knowing and doing, inexperienced instructors often do not understand the importance of these attitudes in determining the outcomes of treatment. Videotapes that show the strengths and weaknesses of different teaching styles may be useful in enabling residents to develop a manner that resonates with students.

Presentations on rounds should be brief – two minutes or less – and include the diagnosis, an update on the patient's condition, pertinent physical findings, and a statement of what is planned and why. When the diagnosis is known, as with most orthopaedic admissions, discussion centers on management and supporting data. Resident comment should be limited to one or two key points, with emphasis on relevance rather than completeness.

Teaching in the operating room is focused on applied anatomy and provides students with a unique opportunity for correlation of pathologic, clinical, laboratory, and radiographic findings. Open-ended questions, such as the importance of a particular finding, the options and rationale for management of a given problem, and the correlation of clinical with laboratory findings are useful means to deepen discussion in all arenas.

Whatever the venue, the medical student should be made to feel an integral and essential member of the health care team, with roles and responsibilities commensurate with his or her knowledge and skill.

4 Absence of service-specific learning objectives for clinical clerks
  There should be clearly stated behavioral objectives for the musculoskeletal education of medical students. For those doing clinical rotations in surgical fields, these objectives should include

the knowledge and skills they are expected to master in the operating room, as well as those in the clinic and at the bedside.

Before their appearance on the floors or in the clinics, students and residents should be made aware of the learning objectives for students on that rotation. When stated in behavioral and measurable terms, objectives guide teaching and evaluation. In addition to the requirements for possession, comprehension, and application of requisite knowledge, objectives should include skills (motor and interactive) and attitudes. The latter are more difficult to construct and to teach, but are ultimately of greater importance. Upon completion of the rotation, students should evaluate the teaching effectiveness of residents.

5 Lack of institutional and/or departmental recognition for excellence in student teaching
Resident teaching is too seldom monitored, supervised, or evaluated, which does not encourage resident effort in this area. The departmental commitment to resident teaching can be made evident by workshops staffed by a faculty member and an educational specialist to improve the teaching skills and confidence of residents.[15]

The value placed on teaching should be further emphasized by including on rating forms a category that rates the resident's effectiveness as a teacher, with special recognition for those who achieve high ratings.

6 Lack of interest in teaching
Residents who like to teach are usually rated favorably on teaching ability, although the extent to which an interest in teaching is innate as opposed to acquired is unclear.[1] Most people, however, enjoy doing things they do well, which justifies our efforts to make even uninterested residents better teachers – as we continue to search in the selection process for ways to identify applicants with a genuine desire to teach. House officers who enjoy working with students will be more likely to involve them and to make themselves accessible, attributes that garner high marks from learners.[1]

Year-end excellence in teaching awards should recognize residents as well as faculty.

Finally, we must stress to deans and educational policy committees the need for mission-based fiscal support of faculty with defined educational responsibilities; and national medical organizations should petition all levels of government for strong and continuous support of graduate medical education.

There is perhaps no better conclusion to this chapter than the statement of Sir William Osler who, over 100 years ago, said, "I desire no other epitaph . . . than the statement that I taught medical students on the wards, as I regard this as by far the most useful and important work I have been called upon to do."[16]

REFERENCES

1 Bing-You RG, Harvey BJ. Factors related to residents' desire and ability to teach in the clinical setting. *Teach Learn Med*. 1991; **3**: 95–100.

2 Bing-You RG, Tooker J. Teaching skills improvement programs in US internal medicine residencies. *Med Educ*. 1993; **27**(3): 259–65.

3 Wilson FC. Residents as teachers. *J Bone Joint Surg Am*. 2001; **83**(9): 1441–3.

4 Brown RS. House staff attitudes toward teaching. *J Med Educ*. 1970; **45**(3): 156–9.

5 Rotenberg BW, Woodhouse RA, Gilbart M, *et al*. A needs assessment of surgical residents as teachers. *Can J Surg*. 2000; **43**(4): 295–300.

6 Sheets KJ, Hankin FM, Schwenk TL. Preparing surgery house officers for their teaching role. *Am J Surg*. 1991; **161**(4): 443–9.

7 Stenchever MA, Irby D, O'Toole B. A national survey of undergraduate teaching in obstetrics and gynecology. *J Med Educ*. 1979; **54**(6): 467–70.

8 Griffith CH 3rd, Georgesen JC, Wilson JF. Specialty choices of students who actually have choices: the influence of excellent clinical teachers. *Acad Med*. 2000; **75**(4): 278–82.

9 Nutter DO, Bond JS, Coller BS, *et al.* Measuring faculty effort and contributions in medical education. *Acad Med.* 2000; **75**(2): 199–207.

10 Pardes H. The perilous state of academic medicine. *JAMA.* 2000; **283**(18): 2427–9.

11 Morrison EH, Rucker L, Boker JR, *et al.* The effect of a 13-hour curriculum to improve residents' teaching skills: a randomized trial. *Ann Intern Med.* 2004; **141**(4): 257–63.

12 Wipf JE, Orlander JD, Anderson JJ. The effect of a teaching skills course on interns' and students' evaluation of their resident–teachers. *Acad Med.* 1999; **74**(8): 938–42.

13 Mass S, Shah SS, Daly SX, *et al.* Effect of feedback on obstetrics and gynecology residents' teaching performance and attitudes. *J Reprod Med.* 2001; **46**(7): 669–74.

14 Whitman N. *Creative Medical Teaching.* Salt Lake City, UT: University of Utah School of Medicine; 1990.

15 Spickard A 3rd, Corbett EC Jr, Schorling JB. Improving residents' teaching skills and attitudes toward teaching. *J Gen Intern Med.* 1996; **11**(8): 475–80.

16 Osler W. The fixed period. Valedictory address at Johns Hopkins Hospital. *JAMA.* 1905; **44**: 705–10.

10

Mentoring Young Physicians

The Need for Nurture*

In Homer's *Odyssey*, Mentor, an old and trusted friend, was left by Odysseus in charge of his house, in which capacity Mentor (or Athena disguised as Mentor) guided the growth and development of Telemachus, Odysseus' son, for the 20 years that Odysseus spent fighting in and returning from the Trojan War. Historically then, mentoring was an extended relationship between a protégé and a more experienced and wiser friend. While Mentor was a remarkably sagacious advisor, his personal investment makes clear that this quality lies at the heart of successful mentoring.

Mentoring may be defined as a relationship, formal and/or informal, between a novice and one or more senior persons in the field for the purposes of career and personal development.

This topic has received wide attention in the corporate world, where benefits of mentoring have been shown in job satisfaction, personal and professional development, higher wages, and employee retention. Seventy-six percent of *Fortune* Magazine's 100 best companies to work for in America offer mentoring programs, compared to 56% of the rest.[1]

---

*   Published in a slightly different version as "Mentoring in orthopaedics: an evolving need for nurture" *Journal of Bone and Joint Surgery*. 2004; **86**(5): 1089–91. It appears here with the permission of that Journal.

Mentoring in medicine has usually consisted of an informal relationship between an established scientist and a young physician-scientist to develop the research capability of the junior investigator. Increasingly sophisticated research and rapid evolution of the health care system have led to expansion of this dyadic model to include a network of colleagues that cross institutional and geographic boundaries – a college without walls.

In times of rapid and profound change, as those occurring now in medicine, mentoring is crucial for the development of physicians who can meet these challenges. More than role modeling is needed, although the amount and type of professional and personal support required by young physicians will vary according to person, age, specialty, type of practice, gender, and career goals. A report from the University of North Carolina at Chapel Hill School of Medicine, for which all departmental chairs and 84 tenure-track junior faculty members were interviewed and completed a questionnaire, indicated a clearly-defined need for mentoring of young physicians, particularly in the areas of research and departmental and institutional policies. Other topics thought to be essential for developing and managing a productive career were outcome-based practice patterns, informatics, and a reconsideration of human values.[2]

ISSUES AND OPTIONS

There are at least six obstacles to developing productive mentoring programs:

1 A culture that does not favor seeking help
   Professional neophytes, especially those in medical fields, are often unwilling to admit that they need help or have problems. They are skilled, knowledgeable, and older than those who embark on business careers. Further, the culture of medicine is authoritative; physicians expect to direct an encounter rather than to be directed.

   For those unwilling to admit the need for help, recognition by the chair that they are *expected* to have problems, and that acknowledging them is a sign of strength rather than weakness, is reassuring. Those who aspire to leadership in the field must realize the value of associations with people who have been there and done that; they must see and hear leaders in their own and other fields so that they may better understand and deal with broader and evolving medical and cultural issues.

For young investigators searching for grant information and/or collaborators, a valuable resource may be their discipline's research society, some of which have mentoring committees to facilitate the careers of neophyte scientists by offering services such as grant-writing workshops.

2 Time constraints
Time – an increasingly precious commodity – must be set aside by both mentor and mentee apart from that required for teaching and day-to-day issues.

A formal mentoring affiliation entails meetings at least quarterly for the first year when participants are free of other duties to allow sufficient time for full discussion of professional and personal issues. For productive sessions, preliminary preparation by both parties is essential. Without such commitment, mentoring relationships often deteriorate into hit-and-run, question-and-answer encounters or die completely from neglect.

It should be further understood that if the relationship is not working, either party can request an alternative partner without recrimination.

Where long-distance mentoring support is needed, a web-based approach may be useful.[3] Such systems allow both mentee and mentor to enter data defining their needs and skill sets, and allow coordinators to monitor progress and measure success. Both formal and informal programs are available and greatly reduce the time required for programmatic development and coordination.

3 Lack of skills for mentoring professional development
No one person can provide all needed support at each stage of another's professional development. New physicians need help

with local policies, politics, and expectations; later, developing a research program and writing grants may become priorities; and for those who become interested in generic issues and professional associations, leadership skills may become necessary.

The professional skills of mentors can be improved by workshops and symposia covering such topics as the matching of mentors and mentees, the formulation of a written academic development plan with short- and long-term goals, defining the academic skills needed by mentees, the writing of grants and scientific papers, curriculum development, and the level and type of support needed from the department and institution.

Because of the diverse and evolving needs of young physicians, mentors must be able and willing to put mentees in contact with secondary mentors who can deal with needs that lie outside their own areas of interest or experience.

4 Lack of skills for mentoring personal development
Good mentors ask thoughtful questions and avoid imposing their own beliefs on mentees. Cloning is not a goal. They must be able to think outside the box of focal medical knowledge and technology in favor of broader issues and differing goals and lifestyles. Their role is to inspire and encourage analytic thought – emphasizing "why" over "how." Those who know how will always have work to do; the person who *directs* their effort will be one who understands why.

The interpersonal aspects of mentoring are critical. Mentors must be committed both to the concept of mentoring and to the mentee. Mentoring includes teaching, advising, and serving as role models, but a good mentor is more than that. Good mentors bring to the table the experience of an examined life. They must be creative listeners who encourage and enable mentees to find their own path, using questions and empathy more than direction – remembering that mentors are not all-knowing, and that their own solutions or suggestions may not be as well suited for persons with different backgrounds, personalities, or gender. One size does not fit everyone.

5 Lack of institutional support

The absence of visible reinforcement from chairs and key institutional personnel critically impairs the effectiveness of mentoring programs. In the academic setting, it is probably unwise, however, for the chair of a department to be a primary mentor, since he or she is directly involved with assessment, promotion, and salary considerations. Formal mentoring can become counterproductive if mentors also assume roles as supervisors and/or assessors.

In addition to clear and ongoing support of time, effort, and process, the senior associate or departmental chair, as part of the orientation for new faculty and residents, should make clear the expectation that each will select a primary mentor, usually within the department, for which brief biographical sketches that include special areas of interest and experience are made available.

6 Other potential problems

Random assignment of mentees to conscripted mentors produces "forced friendships," which, like blind dates, sometimes work out and sometimes do not. Personality clashes, failure to establish core values as a basis for career planning, and unrealistic expectations may also result in unsuccessful mentoring.

The first few sessions are crucial to the success of any mentoring relationship, especially if the partners are of different genders or ethnicities, or there is a large age gap. Establishment and regular review of core values and career plans are essential, although – as with all goal-setting – strict adherence to initial goals is unnecessary if more vital priorities arise. Early in the course of the meetings, both parties, along with assurance of confidentiality, should discuss realistic expectations and limitations for the relationship. Personality clashes or mismatched goals and interests must be recognized early and corrected by reassignment.

Mentoring partnerships in medicine need not be permanent relationships. They are intended to support professional integration without long-term obligations from either party, although such associations are often continued informally as the mentee continues to develop his or her career and to utilize other resources both in and beyond institutional boundaries.

REFERENCES

1 The 100 best companies to work for in America. *Fortune*. January 10, 2000.

2 Granger N, Frey JJ, Gray MJ, *et al.* Mentoring and faculty development: is there a need for nurturing? *A Report of the Committee on Faculty Development and Affirmative Action*. Chapel Hill, NC: University of North Carolina at Chapel Hill School of Medicine; 1993.

3 Corporate Mentoring Solutions, Inc. Available at: www.mentoring-resources.com.

11

Funding Graduate
Medical Education

Who Will Pay?*

Most proposals for the reform of health care delivery have focused
on issues of cost control, access, and quality; relatively few have addressed the education of physicians. Over time, however, the size
and quality of the health care system depends on maintaining an
adequate work force.

Undergraduate medical education is funded from state and local
sources, federal grants and contracts, hospital support, student tuition, and clinical outcome. Financing sources for the costs of GME
are more limited, relying in large part on the Medicare program and
on Medicaid in many states, with the residual costs being funded
out of private insurance patient care dollars. Given the primacy of
Medicare funding, governmental proposals to reduce Medicare funding sent tremors through academic institutions.

The Medicare program, enacted in 1965, provided partial funding
for the education of trainees as an element in the cost of medical care,
pointing out that:

Educational activities enhance the quality of care in an institution, and it
is intended, until the community undertakes to bear such education costs

---

*   In preparing this chapter, I have relied heavily on the resources of the Association
    of American Medical Colleges, whose cooperation is gratefully acknowledged.

in some other way, that a part of the net cost of such activities (including stipends of trainees, as well as compensation of teachers and other costs) should be considered as an element in the cost of patient care, to be borne to an appropriate extent by the hospital insurance program.[1]

This prescient action created a reliable revenue stream for resident education until 1995, at which time, stimulated by the drain on Medicare produced by increasing resident numbers and salaries, voices in Congress began to question and recommend changes in this method of funding GME.[2]

Medicare is the major single source of support for the unique costs of teaching hospitals. It does so primarily through two mechanisms: direct graduate medical education (DGME) offsets, and the indirect medical education (IME) adjustment. DGME funds offset graduate education costs – primarily salaries and benefits of residents and supervising faculty – while indirect payments support the higher costs of patient care resulting from the presence of teaching programs.

From 1965 to 1985, DGME reimbursements were open-ended, with the Medicare program paying its share of any increase in a hospital's increased DGME costs.

With passage of the Consolidated Omnibus Budget Reconciliation Act (COBRA) in 1986, Congress changed the DGME payment methodology, first by establishing hospital-specific per resident amounts, and second, by limiting the number of years of full support to the number of years required for initial board certification. For additional training, DGME payments were reduced to 50%.[3]

The calculation of DGME payments begins with each hospital's cost per resident in a base year, generally 1984, updated to the current year for inflation, which is known as the "per resident amount." The per resident amount is then multiplied by the number of residents in the current year and then by the hospital's ratio of Medicare inpatient days to total days. Because of this ratio, Medicare does not pay for the full GME costs, but only its "share." DGME payments in fiscal year 2008 were estimated at $2.7 billion.[4]

Since passage of the COBRA, Congressional debates and legislation over Medicare DGME payments have focused on a variety of issues, including payments for ambulatory training, differential payments for primary care versus nonprimary care residents, and limits on the variation in per resident amounts. However, probably the most significant change since the COBRA was in the Balanced Budget Act (BBA) of 1997, which capped the number of residents who can be counted for either DGME or IME payments. The law states that for Medicare support, a hospital's number of residents may not exceed the number reported on the hospital's most recent cost report that ended on or before December 31, 1996. The cap on resident physicians generated little concern in 1996 because of the perception that the U.S. was on the verge of an oversupply of physicians. The notation that no definitive conclusions could be drawn about the supply of physicians in 2002 was followed in 2006 by the recognition that there was a physician shortage, and that medical schools should increase their enrollment 30% over 2002 levels by 2015.[5,6] If realized, the increase would require expansion in the number of residency positions to produce more practitioners.

A law that created floors and ceilings for hospital per resident payments addressed the issue of variation in per resident reimbursement rates. Beginning in 2001, a hospital's per resident allocation was adjusted if it was below 70% or above 140% of the national per resident average adjusted for locality. If the hospital's per resident payment was between 70% and 140%, it continued at current levels, updated annually by the CPI increase. In 2002, the floor was raised from 70% to 85%, with no change in the 140% ceiling. As a result of these changes, over 500 of the 1100 hospitals that provide GME received increased DGME payments.[7]

The indirect medical education (IME) adjustment is a payment associated with each Medicare inpatient discharge. It is based on the realization that teaching hospitals have inherently higher costs related to sicker patients, serve as referral centers for other hospitals, and support education and research.

IME costs, in contrast to those for DGME, are less precisely quantifiable. Since they are included among the costs of inpatient care, they must be estimated through regression analyses, which for fiscal 2008 were $5.7 billion.[4]

The IME payment formula uses intern and resident-to-bed (IRB) ratios and a nationwide adjustment factor, which varies from year to year. As a rule of thumb, however, teaching hospitals receive about a 5.5% increase in Medicare per case payments for every 10-resident increase per 100 beds. In other words, the greater the educational "intensity," the higher the IME adjustment.[8]

IME payments have been the subject of considerable debate and legislation. As with DGME reimbursement, there is a "cap" on the number of residents that can be included in the IRB ratio, which is based on how many residents the hospital was training in 1996. Another key focus has been the national adjustment factor. Since 1997, the factor has been legislatively reduced nearly 30% on the premise that the adjustment is higher than statistical analysis suggests it should be.

While Medicare is the largest explicit payer for the special missions of teaching hospitals, state Medicaid programs also offset teaching hospitals' mission-related costs. In fiscal 2005, Medicaid payments for DGME and IME were approximately $3.2 billion.[9] State Medicaid programs are not required to make these additional payments to teaching hospitals, but, recognizing their importance, most states and the District of Columbia have traditionally done so. With many state budgets requiring drastic cutbacks however, Medicaid programs have been targeted for reduced spending, which puts these important teaching-related payments at risk.

Since major teaching hospitals, i.e. those with more than 25 residents for every 100 beds, work on a small profit margin (4.2% in 2005), DGME, IME, and DSH payments are critically important to the fiscal viability of these institutions. The profit margin for nonteaching hospitals in 2005 was 5.2%.[10]

Even though significant, the Medicare and Medicaid funds do not offset fully the mission-related costs at teaching hospitals. Because private payers do not make explicit payments for teaching-related costs, GME costs are offset by portions of the patient care payments teaching hospitals receive.

Before managed care, private insurers simply paid the higher charges submitted by teaching hospitals and faculty for more complex and uninsured patients, as well as for the teaching and research missions.

In the 1980s and 1990s, as *managed care* emerged, this policy changed dramatically. The idea behind managed care was to reduce health care costs by bargaining with providers for the lowest possible cost; as a result, reimbursements to teaching institutions for education and research have decreased steadily.

Cost containment began in earnest when, in 1983, Medicare was ratcheted down by the switch from fee-for-service to *prospective payment*, which established set fees for 467 diagnosis-related groups (DRGs). Private insurers followed, restricting hospital stays and specialist care.[11] Hospitals, to make ends meet, began to stress patient volume. With less time for each patient, quality suffered – as did teaching and research, to which hospitals looked early and often for cuts. Learning opportunities were curtailed. Surgical residents were present for the operative event but had little exposure to equally important preoperative decision-making and postoperative rehabilitation, losing in this compression critical opportunities for patient interactions.

As the institutional focus shifted toward profit margins, the term "Academic Medical Center" (AMC) became something of an oxymoron.[12] With the enormous expansion of clinical activity and the academic mission evolving into the stepchild of practice, AMCs have moved closer to health care systems and away from university ties;[13] however, to the extent that AMCs turn away from universities and toward the health care system, they turn back toward the proprietary schools of the Flexnerian era.

ISSUES AND OPTIONS

Certainly in the several trillion dollars spent annually on health care, support can be found for the education and research needed to ensure the future of medicine.

With the gathering storm forecast for Medicare – kindled by economic recession, exploding health care costs, and an aging population – the need to balance for-profit goals with the teaching and research missions of academic institutions has become urgent.

As with all federal budgets, spending is divided into two main categories: mandatory spending for programs like Medicare and Medicaid, and discretionary or nonmandatory spending for entities such as the National Institutes of Health. One of the most worrisome proposals has been to make DGME payments a discretionary appropriation rather than an entitlement, which would place DGME funding at the indulgence of the same discretionary appropriations as biomedical research. How GME would fare in competition with the National Institutes of Health is problematic, but the uncertainty of funding would undermine stable funding for DGME. It would also introduce the potential for political control by those legislators who want to influence curricular content in residency programs. Even a mandatory appropriation would be subject to similar uncertainties and influences.

Another concern surfaced in the 1999 report of the Medical Payment Advisory Commission (MedPAC), which suggested that DGME and IME costs be combined into a "teaching hospital adjustment," which, since it was intended to produce savings for the Medicare program, would likely reduce current payments for education. The report concluded that Medicare should no longer explicitly support physician training.[14]

A number of organizations, including the AAMC, have supported the creation of a national, "all payer" trust fund to support GME funding and other unique features of teaching hospitals. One 2001–02 legislative proposal required Medicare, Medicaid, and private payer companies to contribute to medical education through a 1.5% assessment on all health insurance premiums.[15] Another suggested continuance of Medicare and Medicaid payments, with the addition of a 1% tax on private health plans. By changing the DGME formula and reducing IME payments, this proposal projected Medicare savings of over a billion dollars annually.[14]

The Medicare Modernization Act (MMA) in 2003 established requirements for submission of both inpatient and outpatient quality-related data, without which a 2% payment reduction would be inflicted, and add-on expenses for preventable complications would not be paid. Hospitals were also required to document value-based purchasing. Further emphasis on efficiency, outcome, and patient safety measures are anticipated for inclusion in this plan.

Given the incipient crisis in Medicare funding, the questions have become "when and how much" rather than "whether" Medicare payments for GME will be decreased. With Congressional budgetary pressures heightened by fiscal recession, the costs of war in the Middle East, Katrina/Rita reconstructions, the prescription drug benefit, and the need for Social Security reform, it is difficult to imagine more Congressional largesse as the complete answer, making the argument for other mechanisms more cogent. Reducing the number of residents – irrational at a time of increasing need – would diminish both the quantity and quality of service that could be provided. Charging tuition, similar to that in other graduate educational programs, would, in effect, reduce the salaries of residents already burdened with loans. Another potential source of added funding, practice income, is shrinking, and endowments would have to be unrealistically large to provide adequate, permanent sources of funding. Requiring remote site affiliated institutions to assume partial responsibility for the costs of education received by residents *prior* to their service in the affiliate is an option that could be explored.

Commitment to GME should also be manifest at the departmental level. While clinical income cannot bear the full costs of GME, using it to enrich educational programs and support resident research, benefits these programs and justifies solicitation from other sources. To achieve academic departmental goals, faculty must be willing to sacrifice part of their personal compensation. Detsky and Baker have described a successful departmental practice plan to achieve these objectives, which includes: 1) pooling of departmental income; 2) a base salary for each faculty member based on job description; 3) an academic bonus based on defined academic productivity; 4) an income bonus based on income contribution, with predetermined targets based on job description; 5) a percentage of overage to the department; 6) development of clear, but not immutable, guidelines; and 7) establishment of an oversight committee.[15]

Whether Medicare is extended, other sources found, and/or costs (and service) cut, stable funding for the GME enterprise must be assured. AMCs, for their part, must acknowledge their commitment to the public by producing enough physicians to meet burgeoning societal needs of growth, diversity, aging, and chronic disease, which will entail producing more generalists (especially geriatricians), greater educational emphasis on quality of care, prevention, and efficiency, and an intensified research focus on diseases and disorders that have major health care implications.

REFERENCES

1 House Report, Number 213, 89th Congress. 1st Sess. (1965) and Senate Report, Number 401. Pt 1. 89th Congress. 1st Sess. 36 (1965).

2 Knapp RM. Complexity and uncertainty in financing graduate medical education. *Acad Med.* 2002; **77**(11): 1076.

3 Knapp, op. cit. p. 1077.

4 Harris H, Gabriel BA. Graduate medical education and health care reform. *Reporter.* 2009; **18**(10): 5.

5 Knapp, op. cit. p. 1078.

6 *AAMC Statement on the Physician Workforce.* Washington, DC: Association of American Medical Colleges; 2005.

7 Knapp, op. cit. p. 1079.

8 Knapp, op. cit. p. 1080.

9 Henderson TM. Medicaid direct and indirect graduate medical education payments: a 50-state survey. Washington, DC: Association of American Medical Colleges; Nov 2006, p. 6.

10 *Medicare Payment Advisory Commission Databook.* Washington, DC: MedPAC; June 2007.

11 Ludmerer KM. *Time to Heal: American medical education from the turn of the century to the era of managed care.* Oxford: Oxford University Press; 1999. p. 351.

12 Ludmerer, op. cit. p. 367.

13 Ludmerer, op. cit. p. 336.

14 Knapp, op. cit. p. 1082.

15 Detsky AS, Baker MA. How to run a successful academic practice plan. *JAMA.* 2007; **298**(7): 799–801.

12

Manpower
Supply and Distribution

ISSUES AND OPTIONS

Closely related to the funding of GME are issues of resident numbers and their distribution by specialty and location – which determine the size, mix, and deployment of the physician work force. In addition to shrinking physician-to-population ratios and the maldistribution of doctors by specialty and geography, other determinants also complicate manpower needs and projections: gender and generational issues, IMGs and the migration of physicians into the U.S., variation in the use and efficiency of medical services, the role of nonphysician providers, and the surge in demand produced by an aging population.[1]

Given the number and complexity of manpower problems, it is not surprising that there is no single, simple solution. Complex problems require complex solutions. Univariate answers to multivariate questions are unfailingly misleading.

With specialty choices determined largely by issues of income and lifestyle, fewer students are choosing careers in primary care. High-tech specialties offer exciting opportunities for cure; but older patients, having chronic conditions, are often more in need of care than cure – for someone to be there, to guide them through the complex world of health care, and to manage multiple diseases and depression. Despite the fact that most of the problems for which a physician is consulted can be handled by generalists, they have become an endangered species. Unless the Millennial Generation is less self-serving and materialistic than Generation X, the scene of a personal physician sitting by a patient's bedside may come to exist only in a Luke Fildes painting.

Although criticized by the Office of Management and Budget for lack of effectiveness and not producing specific outcomes, Title VII, Section 747 Programs have, since their inception in 1972, contributed significantly to the development of primary care and physician assistant (PA) training to provide health care for disadvantaged populations. Sharpening the focus and establishing specific, measurable, outcome parameters would justify refunding of these programs (cost to date $3.9 billion in 2008 dollars).[2]

Bell, *et al.* have suggested an accelerated medical school curriculum to promote careers in primary care. Students who meet certain academic standards are admitted to medical school after three years of college and attend medical school essentially year-round for three years, with two-week "vacations" at the end of the first and second years. They complete the core clinical rotations in the third year and eliminate "redundant and minimally effective audition rotations" in the fourth year. With career paths determined, additional time for decision-making is unnecessary. All students in the primary care track have faculty mentors assigned upon entry to medical school, and the teaching roles of primary care physicians are expanded by their inclusion in other courses and clerkships. The effectiveness of this approach is being assessed as experience accumulates.[3]

Halvorsen has recommended unification of the primary care disciplines into a single specialty, pointing out that the U.S. is the only industrialized Western nation that provides primary care by means of a fragmented system. Consolidation of Internal Medicine, Family Medicine, and Pediatrics – currently separated by a common goal – would give primary care a single, powerful voice nationally, promote the formation of integrated primary care teams, and facilitate development of a primary care "home" for every American. By merging training in these disciplines, with common curricula and standards, the education of both medical students and residents could be enhanced, and health care delivery made more efficient and less costly.[4]

As Kirch pointed out, the best approach to strengthening primary care is at the beginning, with a collaborative, high-quality educational program rather than beginning at the other end of the spectrum with "work force shaping." He suggests the medical home concept with new models of reimbursement and delivery as one means to achieve coordination and continuity of health care.[5]

The American Academy of Pediatrics, the American College of Physicians, and the American Academy of Family Physicians endorsed the medical home project to improve the delivery of health care with a statement of joint principles in March 2007, which the AAMC has adopted: each person should have access to a medical home with a designated provider to serve as the point of first contact; further testing is necessary to determine the optimal means for implementation and performance assessment; payment should recognize and reward health care providers appropriately for their contribution to prevention and coordination as well as care; education is needed, particularly for specialists and nonphysician providers; and academic health centers should be involved to provide capital and operational support for establishing medical homes in larger communities.[6]

The call for testing of the Patient-Centered Medical Home Model has been authorized in the Medicare Medical Home Demonstration Project embedded in the Tax Relief and Health Care Act of 2006. It authorizes several demonstration projects in the U.S. that involve commercial payers, Medicaid agencies, national employers, business groups, medical specialty societies, and health services researchers. Of course, implementing this model for all Medicare beneficiaries would make balancing an overburdened Medicare budget even more difficult, probably entailing cost sharing by beneficiaries and reducing payments to physicians and hospitals.

Although primary care specialties and the AMA have not looked with favor on the proliferation of convenient care clinics based in retail stores and staffed by PAs and nurse practitioners, our inability to meet the health care needs for a rapidly expanding and diverse population makes "retail medicine" a partial and currently necessary alternative to the shortage of primary care physicians.[7] By improving access to care and lowering costs, it addresses two major problems confronting American health care. The 70 000 PAs practicing under the supervision of a physician are growing annually at 5%, which, if continued, will double the number of PAs by 2020.[8]

Whether reliance on International Medical Graduates (some 25% of the physician workforce) should be increased to fill gaps in specialty and geographic distribution is less clear, since to the extent that we rely on outside help, we are failing to meet our own needs. Clearly, however, the provision of waivers for all physicians with J-1 visas for service in areas of demand would allow them to remain in this country, even if they leave after two or three years.

Service in the National Health Service Corps, which provides loan repayment for practice in underserved areas, also addresses the geographic distribution of physicians. It is a proven and valuable program that deserves expansion, even to the point of requiring a period of service in areas of need as the *quid pro quo* for students who receive federal loans.

With the current emphasis on competency, it may also be a propitious time for GME to move to a competency-based model rather than specific time requirements, which would, for many residents, shorten the length of training.

REFERENCES

1 Kirch DG, Vernon DJ. Confronting the complexity of the physician workforce equation. *JAMA*. 2008; **299**(22): 2680–2.

2 Reynolds PP. Why we need to restore primary care generalist training as the centerpiece of federal policy. *Acad Med*. 2008; **83**(11): 993–5.

3 Bell HS, Ferretti SM, Ortoski RA. A three-year accelerated medical school curriculum designed to encourage and facilitate primary care careers. *Acad Med*. 2007; **82**(9): 895–9.

4 Halvorsen JG. United we stand, divided we fall: the case for a single primary care specialty in the United States. *Acad Med*. 2008; **83**(5): 425–31.

5 Kirch DG. The primary care "crisis." *AAMC Reporter*. 2008; **18**(1): 2.

6 *The Medical Home: AAMC position statement*. Washington, DC: Association of American Medical Colleges; February 2008.

7 Moskowitz EJ. Retail medicine. *Health Policy Newsletter*. Jefferson Medical College, Sept 2007; **20**(3): 1–2.

8 Barwick TA, Lane S. PAs: not a silent partner. *AAMC Reporter*. 2009; **18**(4): 3.

13

Obligations of Residents
With Rights Come Responsibilities

In their requirements for accreditation, the ACGME has defined the institutional obligations to residents. A successful partnership is more likely, however, when both parties benefit, so residents must understand and fulfill their obligations to the institutions in which they serve.

There are at least seven groups of people to whom house officers are responsible: their patients, their families, society, institutional personnel, fellow residents, students, and self. These comments will focus on groups related to the institution: faculty, administrators, patients, nurses, other residents and students.

ISSUES AND OPTIONS
The complex, generic issues in graduate medical education – funding, subspecialization, and maldistribution among them – will require intervention at the national level; but there are many things residents can do to minimize institutional problems, beginning with resisting the temptation to complain and criticize. Hospital policies exist not because they are the best answer for each resident, but because they represent the best compromise for all. There is much in the life of a resident – or any life – to find fault with; but criticism should be constructive, going beyond recognition of the problem to a solution – and one that does not cause more problems than it solves.

Residents are, in large part, responsible for the quality of the physicians who come after them. Junior residents, presuming that senior residents have been successful, will pattern their behavior accordingly, which emphasizes the importance of role modeling by those who have succeeded.

There will also be times when a resident should think not in terms of his or her job, but of the job that needs doing – when things will run more safely or efficiently if a resident functions temporarily as nurse, secretary, or member of the transportation team. National shortages in nursing make this an especially critical area for good working relationships.

Hospital records, often the only source of critical medical information, rely heavily on residents' findings and actions, which should be recorded accurately, concisely, and promptly.

Resident participation on institutional committees, cumbersome as it may be, is often the best way to work toward solutions of problems that cannot be resolved by individual interactions.

In contacts with patients and their families, residents should avoid medical jargon, remembering that patients are people, not physicians; and that, irrespective of gender, race, religion, or economic status, they should be treated with dignity and respect. It is disturbing to hear a resident greet an 80-year-old patient as "Honey." They have names that should be remembered and used; however, it is patronizing for a physician to introduce himself as "Dr. Jones," while addressing a much older patient as "Barbara." Given the importance of a sense of equality in human relations, such asymmetries of address are demeaning and suggest power imbalances, which makes common ground difficult to establish.

There is an understandable tendency for doctors to be authoritarian in their dealings with patients, but good physicians encourage patient involvement, which entails getting to know them and their circumstances. Until its recognition as one of the core competencies, medical education had given little formal attention to communication skills, regarding them as a by-product of content mastery. Of course, knowing one's patients does not insure liking them, but a negative reaction may, unless recognized and suppressed, affect management adversely.

Although a shotgun approach to ordering diagnostic studies may benefit education (and occasionally patient care), cost has become a major player in these decisions; and, since fiscal constraints are likely to increase, improvements must be found in greater efficiency, better organization, and innovation rather than more tests or analyses.

Finally, residents should ask for help when help is needed. Residents are residents because they do not possess the requisite knowledge and skills for optimal patient care. One of the best indicators of an insecure or incompetent resident is a reluctance to seek advice.

The faculty will expect residents to be reliable, prepared, and on time; and to bear in mind that the learner more than the teacher determines the level of educational achievement. The faculty and institution provide guidance and a learning environment, but residents must be the primary stewards of their own education.

In dealings with peers and students, the rule is teach, teach, teach. The word "doctor," derived from the Latin *docere*, means "to teach." Residents as well as faculty have that obligation to other health care personnel. All of us owe much to many for our own education; it is a debt that cannot be paid back but can be paid forward.

At the heart of all medical encounters is professionalism. If residents expect to be treated as professionals, they must be professional in dress, demeanor, and deportment as well as competence. An unkempt appearance and joking with staff or peers are generally not well received by patients who often assume they are the subjects of disrespect or mirth.

These suggestions are not comprehensive. They were chosen to remind residents of their responsibilities for making education a two-way street. If there is give as well as take, they will grow as professionals, enriching the institution as well as themselves.

14

Recommendations
What Then Must We Do?

Fitting the many, disparate pieces of the GME puzzle into a single, immutable paradigm for progress is neither feasible nor desirable. Shifting demographics and perceptions of need are changing the size and shape of even the commonalities in a system increasingly characterized by diversity.

Many of the problems in GME can and should be addressed at the departmental or institutional level. Others will require support from national organizations and legislative bodies. What follows is a list of specific suggestions for change, with the rationale for each. Rather than attempting to arrange these recommendations in order of importance, they follow the sequence in which these topics were covered in earlier sections of the book.

CREDENTIALING
Recommendation #1: *The ACGME must, in accredited programs, support promising innovation and experimentation designed to improve resident performance.*

To accomplish this goal, the ACGME may need to relax current standards and requirements, as, for example, for a proposal to alter the educational requirements in a given program. This effort will require close coordination between program directors, certifying boards, and the ACGME.

Recommendation #2: *The process of accreditation must be streamlined to reduce complexity, increase efficiency, and improve communication with program directors.*

Since a visit by the RRC commonly requires several months of preparation by the program director and staff, the elimination of paper forms and reduction of program information requirements by the ACGME are central to this objective.

Instructional programs offered by the ACGME for new program directors would reduce communication gaps, misunderstandings, and errors in reporting.

TEACHING AND LEARNING

Recommendation #3: *As quality control standards and measures are established, a user-friendly, interactive communication system with access to centralized databases must be available in health care centers.*

The use of web-based information technology will, by reducing the time and effort currently required to gather and integrate data, improve clinical decision-making at the point of contact – and thus resident education. It will also facilitate clinical research by reducing the work currently required for manual and/or spreadsheet data collection and chart review.

Recommendation #4: *Medicine's underlying values and goals must be emphasized throughout the educational experience, beginning in the baccalaureate years.*

Medical education has stressed the acquisition of scientific and technical knowledge, but given insufficient attention to the humanistic and cultural values that should determine its use. The values on which medicine is based – competence, altruism, integrity, and empathy – should be reaffirmed and emphasized, since they will determine the plane upon which medicine is practiced.

Premedical education should be reconfigured to produce a better balance between the physical and social sciences and the liberal arts to enhance responsiveness to issues of cultural and social diversity that students, residents, and practitioners encounter on a daily basis. An education in the liberal arts expands the window through which one views life. Too often, we fail to take advantage of the baccalaureate years to broaden the base for building a life in medicine. Understanding promotes empathy, which promotes caring. Literature and art add vicarious understanding of the human predicament; so, in addition to teaching the art of medicine, perhaps we should, through discussions of illness in painting and literature, teach the medicine of art.

Recommendation #5: *All disciplines must establish learning objectives and opportunities focused on resident performance in each of the six competency domains defined by the ACGME.*

The curriculum for such programs should include behavioral objectives, teaching methodology, and a valid, reliable, and practical plan for measuring achievement – even though adequate performance does not ensure a satisfactory clinical result, and outcomes may not be known for years following treatment.

Recommendation #6: *The critical role of residents as teachers must be recognized and strongly supported.*

Institutions and programs should make clear to residents their obligation to teach students and more junior residents. Near-peer teaching relationships are less threatening to learners and offer the teaching resident an opportunity to clarify his/her own thinking without embarrassment. To improve the teaching skills of residents, the department and/or institution should provide instruction to the residents in the principles of adult learning and assessment.

Recommendation #7: *Programs to enhance the educational skills of teaching faculty must be established in each medical school.*

Pedagogic and assessment techniques, principles of curriculum development and mentoring, and educational research methodology should be incorporated in a program or fellowship for those faculty members in each department who wish to make education a major part of their academic careers.

EVALUATION

Recommendation #8: *Each discipline must include professional judgment among its parameters of evaluation as a source of qualitative information for resident assessment.*

Judgments by experienced professionals are often the best source of information for performance evaluation, especially in the affective domain. Objective assessment relies largely upon standardized measurement of specified content; however, with adequate sampling, reliability can also be achieved with subjective evaluation.[1]

Recommendation #9: *Assessment in practice settings and simulations must be endorsed by the ACGME as a substantive component of resident evaluation.*

Since content validity is a function of how well the evaluation measures what it is purported to measure, progress toward measurement authenticity is important, with its optimal end point being testing in real world contexts. Reliable methods of practice-based assessment are emerging that allow evaluation of practice performance through ascending levels from *knowing* to knowing *how* (computer simulations), to *showing* how (performance simulations, as with the OSCE), to habitual *performance* in practice (Miller's pyramid).[1]

Recommendation #10: *Each specialty must develop well-defined, standardized, competency-based curricula for resident education, upon which educational offerings and certifying examinations are based.*

Specified curricular objectives focus the teaching program and provide content validity for certifying examinations.

Recommendation #11: *The ACGME must continue its efforts to develop more valid and reliable methods to assess resident performance.*

Medical knowledge is an important determinant of the quality of patient care. Its presence does not ensure that it will be used, but its absence assures that it will not, which justifies continued efforts to improve the validity and reliability of certifying examinations.

As experience accumulates, the ACGME should provide increasingly specific guidelines for program directors to improve assessment of the core competencies, especially those components in the affective domain.

PROFESSIONALISM

Recommendation #12: *Professionalism must be taught formally in each phase of medical education.*

By giving professionalism formal curricular attention, young physicians are likely to focus more critically on their ethical obligations to patients, peers, and society in subsequent clinical interactions.

Professionalism is not just a philosophical ideal, nor can it be marginalized by the need for efficiency or productivity. It should be defined according to its characteristic traits, its cognitive base made clear, and opportunities provided to gain experience in its application to daily medical care. Many of its basic principles, e.g. ethics and morality, could be explored in premedical philosophy courses.

Teaching opportunities during medical school and residency include lectures, direct observation, simulations and role modeling. The latter is especially critical, since learners will follow what teachers and mentors do rather than what they say. Patient interviews, 360 degree evaluations, and objective, self-reflective comments in portfolios are methods of assessment that appear promising means to enhance professional growth.

Institutional role modeling is also vital. Medical staff and governing boards must examine their policies on conflict of interest, with particular reference to the pharmaceutical and device industries, retaining those that do not or could not influence medical judgments and eliminating those that do or have the potential to do so. Science, not marketing, should drive health care decisions.

RESEARCH

Recommendation #13: *All residents must be taught the principles of research design, methodology, and validation, and have opportunities to participate in translational/clinical and/or basic research.*

The average age of physicians receiving their first NIH RO1 grant is 43, which emphasizes the need for early and ongoing emphasis on research training.[2]

Research will not be part of every physician's life, but understanding research principles is necessary to evaluate the quality and importance of innovations and findings reported in the medical literature. Early exposure to research will also give future physicians the opportunity to consider incorporating research into their careers. To ensure early contact, the LCME and ACGME must require that programs and institutions provide opportunities for student and resident research in addition to instruction in research principles.

Recommendation #14: *For residents who wish to make translational/clinical investigation a meaningful part of their careers, institutional and departmental support, including funding, protected time, space, and equipment, mentors, and biostatistical consultation must be made available.*

Training residents for translational/clinical research requires close integration and cooperation between the clinical and academic components of Academic Medical Centers. Such programs are valuable because translational research directly benefits teaching and clinical practice. The establishment of local guidelines and support for these programs will undoubtedly make institutions more competitive for extramural funding and resources, such as the NIH's Clinical and Translational Science Awards.

As an additional incentive, the opportunity to obtain a Master's Degree should be available to these trainees, incorporating it into the continuum of medical education so that it will not add more than a year to standard educational requirements.

FUNDING

Recommendation #15: *Stable funding must be found to support residency training, including the additional positions resulting from medical school expansion.*

While the U. S. population has expanded rapidly, the number of residency positions has seen little growth in the past 10 years. Cooper estimated that to produce the 200 000 additional physicians needed in the year 2025, the number of PGY-1 positions would have to be increased by 1000 each year from 2010 to 2020. With the length of residency training averaging over four years, these increments would increase the total number of residents in training by almost 45 000 – a 43% increase – which would narrow but not close the physician supply-demand gap. If these are additional positions, current funding will have to be expanded comparably from government sources (Medicare, Medicaid, and VA), other insurers, clinical practice, and endowment revenues.[3]

Recommendation #16: *Funding for residency education should be obtained primarily through a Medicare-Medicaid entitlement, with preferential funding for new positions in primary care and practice in underserved areas.*

In spite of current congressional ambivalence toward both GME and IME payments, it seems preferable to preserve the traditional central role of Medicare funding rather than to strike out toward another payment system, with its own problems and challenges. The inclusion of private insurers, however, seems only fair and almost certainly will be needed – as will incentives for improving the specialty and geographic distribution of physicians.

MANPOWER: SUPPLY AND DISTRIBUTION

Recommendation #17: *U.S. medical schools must strive to increase enrollment by 30% over 2002 levels by the year 2015.*

With or without unexpected changes in the demand and need for health care and/or practice patterns, substantive increases in medical school capacity are needed.

Even with achievement of this goal, which also requires funding for supplementary faculty, facilities, and residents, it will be another eight years or so before the full complement of added matriculants enter the physician work force, by which time, given a continuously aging and expanding population base, demand will still exceed supply, especially in underserved areas and in geriatric care. For this reason, other approaches, especially those that offer earlier relief, will also be needed.

Recommendation #18: *The 1997 Congressional cap on the number of residents funded by Medicare must be lifted to provide GME positions for projected increases in medical school graduates.*

By 2012, first year enrollments in medical school are projected to increase by 21% over 2002 levels.[4] If student increases are met simply by decreasing the number of IMGs in residency training (most of whom remain in this country), the pool of physicians practicing in the U.S. will not be enlarged significantly, so the number of resident slots, especially in areas of need, must be increased.

Recommendation #19: *Population trends must be studied, and planning for anticipated growth closely coordinated with the capacity of the U.S. health care system for expansion.*

Since resources are finite, and expansion of the physician pool is very costly and time consuming, joint planning by Congress, the LCME, ACGME, and AAMC is essential to meet short- and long-term needs for medical services.

Recommendation #20: *Each phase of medical education must be studied in relation to its subsequent phase to determine how, with better integration and application of new learning theory and informational technology, the time required to educate a physician can be reduced.*

By linking what are now largely independent educational segments as a continuum, curricular gaps and redundancies can be minimized, and the time and costs of medical education diminished. These issues should be deliberated by appropriate national organizations, the LCME, AAMC, ACGME, and ABMS in particular, to determine how premedical, medical, and graduate education can be integrated more effectively to increase the production of physicians, especially those who intend to pursue a primary care track.

Another option that warrants further evaluation is the use of competency standards rather than a set number of years as the basis for determining the length of residency training. Coupled with a reduction in the time spent performing duties that have little or no educational value, it would be possible to reduce the period of GME for most residents.

Recommendation #21: *The National Health Service Corps program must be expanded and funding increased.*

Congressional strengthening of the debt forgiveness program for physicians who practice in underserved areas will address both the geographic and specialty maldistribution of physicians.

Recommendation #22: *The primary care divisions of Internal Medicine and Pediatrics must move toward consolidating their curricula and standards of care with those of Family Medicine to provide a unified primary care discipline for residency training.*

Consolidation of these disciplines would broaden and strengthen primary care and minimize waste, cost, and patient confusion. The major obstacles: loss of specialty identity, organizational issues, and leadership should be addressed by task forces representing the primary care specialties, organized medicine (AAMC, ACGME, ABMS, and AMA), the public, and an appropriate governmental body.

Recommendation #23: *Disciplines, departments, and institutions must increase their emphasis on geriatric education.*

Medical care for the aged drives, and will continue to drive, health care in the U.S. for the foreseeable future. By 2020, some 20% of Americans will be over 65, and people over 85 constitute the most rapidly expanding segment of the population, for which all physicians must be prepared.[4]

Geriatric education must be included in each phase of medical training to ensure that all students and residents develop the fundamental knowledge, skills, and attitudes needed to deal with the tsunamic health care impact of an expanding and aging population. The AAMC-Hartford Geriatric Curricular Program reported the effect of funded ($100 000 per school) efforts by 40 medical schools to develop integrated four-year curricula in geriatrics. Approaches varied among the schools, but the more successful included the use of senior mentors, community partnerships, standardized patients, faculty development programs, computer technology, and curricular emphasis by the institution.[5]

Increased emphasis on geriatrics in medical school should, as a minimum, provide better grounding for the management of specialty-specific geriatric problems in GME.

Recommendation #24: *Reimbursement incentives for generalist care must be brought more in line with those for specialists.*

The lack of financial incentives for primary care disciplines has had a major effect on the career choices of medical students and ultimately on the costs of health care in the U.S. Generalists often deal with multiple problems during an office visit; and the inclusion of preventive measures further prolongs encounter time, which limits the number of patients that can be seen during a given day – and thus the reimbursement.

REFERENCES

1 van der Vleuten CPM, Schuwirth LWT. Assessing professional competence: from methods to programs. *Med Educ.* 2005; **39**(3): 309–17.

2 Reece EA. Averting a gathering storm: research education backstage in medical schools. *AAMC Reporter.* 2008; **17**(12): 3.

3 Cooper RA. It's time to address the problem of physician shortages: graduate medical education is the key. *Ann Surg.* 2007; **246**(4): 527–34.

4 Hampton T. U.S. medical school enrollment rising, but residency programs too limited. *JAMA.* 2008; **299**(24): 2846.

5 Anderson MB, editor. The AAMC-Hartford geriatrics curriculum program: reports from 40 schools. *Acad Med.* 2004; **79**(Suppl. 7): pp. Sv–Sx.

15

Afterword

Having begun this work with a historical fantasy, it seems fitting to close with an imaginary glimpse of the future. The next 25 years, given the incremental rate of change in the 100 years since Flexner, will likely encompass at least comparable alterations in medical education, leading, *unless the trajectory changes*, to:

- A continued preponderance of specialists and subspecialists relative to primary care physicians, with increasing reliance on nonphysician paradigms of general practice.
- More frequent use of computer-assisted instruction, with less reliance on direct student–teacher interactions.
- Less clinical teaching in tertiary care institutions and more in satellite clinics and hospitals.
- Increasing emphasis on noncognitive aspects of performance, especially interpersonal and communication skills.
- Surgical education that is confined largely to the operating room, with more pre- and postoperative care responsibility assumed by primary care physicians and allied health personnel.
- Continued lack of standardized intradisciplinary curricula, with defined performance objectives upon which education and certification examinations are based.
- Less resident involvement with research, especially in laboratory-based investigation.

- Continuing tension between the twin gods of quantity and quality, with the balance favoring quantity.
- Perhaps the greatest impact on learning will result from the accelerating accumulation of internet accessible information in health-related areas. As information technology evolves, sharing of information among clinicians, teachers and learners, and researchers will be the keystone of daily operations. Inevitably, this flow of knowledge will stimulate innovations in teaching and research and new models for the prevention and management of disease. The education of residents will be customized by the availability of cutting-edge knowledge, and interdisciplinary collaboration facilitated by the ease and rapidity of information exchange.

Almost everything will change at some time in some manner. Death and taxes aside, the only certainty is change. Whether academia keeps pace with these changes or regresses to the apprenticeship learning and proprietary hospitals of the Flexnerian era will depend in large measure upon leaders who possess the vision to see, the flexibility to adapt, and a value system that places service to others, education, and innovation in front of financial incentives.

Appendix

Graduate Medical Education Organizations		
Accreditation Council for Graduate Medical Education	ACGME	www.acgme.org
American Board of Medical Specialties	ABMS	www.abms.org
American Hospital Association	AHA	www.aha.org
American Medical Association	AMA	www.ama-assn.org
Council on Medical Education	CME	(312) 464–4649
Fifth Pathway		(312) 464–4666
Find a Residency or Fellowship		(312) 464–4743
GME directory		(312) 464–5333
International Medical Graduates Section	IMG	(312) 464–5622
Resident and Fellow Section		(312) 464–4750
Section on Medical Schools		(312) 464–4655
Association for Hospital Medical Education	AHME	www.ahme.org
Association for the Study of Medical Education	ASME	www.asme.org.uk
Association of Academic Health Centers	AAHC	www.aahcdc.org

Graduate Medical Education Organizations		
Association of American Medical Colleges	AAMC	www.aamc.org
Biomedical and Health Services Research	BHSR	www.aamc.org
Central Group on Educational Affairs	CGEA	www.aamc.org
Coalition for the Advancement of Medical Research	CAMR	www.camradvocacy.org
Competencies across the Continuum of Medical Education	CCME	www.aamc.org
Council of Academic Societies	CAS	www.aamc.org
Council of Deans	COD	www.aamc.org
Council of Teaching Hospitals	COTH	www.aamc.org
Center for Work Force Studies	CWS	www.aamc.org
Electronic Residency Application System (U.S.)	ERAS	www.aamc.org
Foreign medical graduates	FMG	www.aamc.org
Faculty Roster	FR	www.aamc.org
General Professional Education of the Physician	GPEP	www.aamc.org
Group on Educational Affairs	GEA	www.aamc.org
Group on Faculty Affairs	GFA	www.aamc.org
Group on Resident Affairs	GRA	www.aamc.org
Innovations in Medical Education	IME	www.aamc.org
National Resident Matching Program	NRMP	www.nrmp.org
Organization of Resident Representatives	ORR	www.aamc.org
Research in Medical Education	RIME	www.aamc.org
Residency Review Committee	RRC	www.aamc.org
Centers for Medicare and Medicaid Services	CMS	www.cms.hhs.gov
Clinical and Translational Science Award	CTSA	www.nih.gov
Clinical Research Education and Career Development	CRECD	www.nih.gov

Graduate Medical Education Organizations		
Council on Graduate Medical Education	COGME	www.cogme.gov
Council of Medical Specialty Societies	CMSS	www.cmss.org
Department of Health and Human Services	DHHS	www.nih.gov
Educational Commission for Foreign Medical Graduates	ECFMG	www.ecfmg.org
Federal Licensing Examination	FLEX	www.ecfmg.org
Federation of State Medical Boards of the U.S., Inc.	FSMB	www.fsmb.org
Liaison Committee on Medical Education	LCME	www.lcme.org
Medicare Payment Advisory Commission	MEDPAC	www.medpac.gov
National Board of Medical Examiners	NBME	www.nbme.org
National Health Service Corps	NHSC	www.nhsc.hrsa.gov
U.S. Medical Licensing Examination	USMLE	www.usmle.org

Index